VOLUME VIII, NUMBER 4, OCTOBER 2009

CLINICAL UPDATES IN WOMEN'S HEALTH CARE

Care of Aging Women

Morton A. Stenchever, MD
Professor and Chairman Emeritus
Department of Obstetrics
and Gynecology
University of Washington
Medical School
Seattle, Washington

Myron Miller, MD
Professor
Department of Medicine
Johns Hopkins University
School of Medicine
Baltimore, MD

D1397630

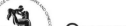

THE AMERICAN COLLEGE OF
OBSTETRICIANS AND GYNECOLOGISTS
WOMEN'S HEALTH CARE PHYSICIANS

Online access for subscribers—www.clinicalupdates.org

Clinical Updates in Women's Health Care is published quarterly by the American College of Obstetricians and Gynecologists. This series represents the knowledge and experience of the authors and does not necessarily reflect the policy of the American College of Obstetricians and Gynecologists. The recommendations do not dictate an exclusive course of treatment or of practice. Variations taking into account the needs of the individual patient, resources, and limitations unique to the institution or type of practice may be appropriate.

ISSN: 1536-3619
ISBN: 978-1-934946-70-1

12345/32109   CU037

Contents

After reading *Care of Aging Women,* go to
www.clinicalupdates.org

- Complete and submit the CME questions online—
  automatically add 5 CME credits to your ACOG
  cognate transcript.
- View links to resources related to the care of aging
  women.
  - American Geriatrics Society
    www.americangeriatrics.org
  - American Psychological Association
    www.apa.org
  - National Institute on Aging
    www.nia.nih.gov
- Order ACOG patient education material
- See full text of past issues and any relevant
  changes or updates

Continuing Medical Education

Objectives
This monograph is designed to enable obstetrician–gynecologists to:

- Understand the effects of the aging process on various organ systems

- Identify common age-associated issues and disorders of women

- Monitor risk factors for various conditions that may occur in older women

- Counsel patients about lifestyle factors, including appropriate nutrition, exercise, and safety precautions, that may improve their quality of life and decrease their risks of morbidity and mortality

- Treat patients for conditions that occur in association with the aging process

- Understand the community resources available and make appropriate referrals both to health care providers and to community services

ACCME Accreditation
The American College of Obstetricians and Gynecologists (ACOG) is accredited by the Accreditation Council for Continuing Medical Education (ACCME) to provide continuing medical education for physicians.

AMA PRA Category 1 Credit™ and ACOG Cognate Credit
The American College of Obstetricians and Gynecologists (ACOG) designates this educational activity for a maximum of 5 AMA PRA Category 1 Credit(s)™ or up to a maximum of 5 Category 1 ACOG cognate credit(s). Physicians should only claim credit commensurate with the extent of their participation in the activity.

Disclosure Statement
Current guidelines state that continuing medical education (CME) providers must ensure that CME activities are free from the control of any commercial interest. All authors and editorial board members declare that neither they nor any business associate nor any member of their immediate families has material interest, financial interest, or other relationships with any company manufacturing commercial products relative to the topics included in this publication or with any provider of commercial services discussed in this publication except for Morton Stenchever, MD, who has financial interests in Merck, Pfizer, Bristol Myers, Wyeth, GlaxoSmithKline, and Amgen and Raul Artal, MD, who has been involved with clinical trials with Nascent, Solvay, Xenodyne, Symbollon Pharmaceuticals, and Columbia Laboratories. Any conflicts have been resolved through group and outside review of all content.

See page iv for submission of CME credits.

Foreword

This monograph, first published in 2004, is designed to provide practitioners with information that will help them to identify and manage medical conditions common in older women. Because obstetrician–gynecologists are providing health care for increasing numbers of older patients, this monograph has been updated to address the changing health care needs of this patient population. Specifically, Myron Miller, MD, an expert geriatrician, provides a perspective from the specialty of geriatrics that broadens the scope of this monograph.

Morton Stenchever, MD
Editor

ABSTRACT. *During the past century, the life expectancy for women has increased from just more than 50 years to more than 80 years. Consequently, women are now postmenopausal approximately one third of their lives. As women age, there is a slow reduction in their physical abilities and a progressive decrease in bone mineralization, muscle mass, cardiopulmonary reserve, microsomal enzyme activity, sensory acuity, and connective tissue integrity. Although knowledge acquired with socialization tends to remain stable in older women, the speed of acquisition and retrieval of new information, creativity, fluidity of thought, and the ability to solve problems decreases. It is important for obstetrician–gynecologists to be aware of how issues such as disease screening; nutrition; exercise; sexuality; immunization; safety; psychologic issues, such as depression, dementia, and grief and loss; domestic violence and abuse; and potential problems of drug interactions are related to the health care needs of their older patients. Additionally, there are many medical conditions that are common in older women that can be managed by obstetrician–gynecologists, such as mild-to-moderate cardiovascular disease and hypertension, incontinence and pelvic floor dysfunction, and vulvar and vaginal conditions.*

In 2004, heart disease was the leading cause of death for women aged 65 years and older (330,513) in the United States, and cancer was the second leading cause of death (267,058) (1). Other major causes of death for women in this age group are stroke (91,274), chronic lower respiratory disease (63,341), Alzheimer disease (46,991), pneumonia and influenza (32,803), diabetes mellitus (37,871), renal disease (22,110), accidents (39,962), and septicemia (18,362).

The objective in providing health care for older women must be to reduce the risk of morbidity and death from the previously mentioned causes and to delay functional decline and dependency for as long as possible. Screening tests for disease should be performed so that acute and chronic illnesses can be detected early. Immunization and disease prophylaxis also should be offered when appropriate. The annual health maintenance examination is an ideal time to address these issues and can be a useful model for promoting good health in older women.

 Basic Science Update

In order to address the changing health care needs of older patients, it is important to understand the processes that contribute to changes in health. Knowledge of the theories of aging and the development of frailty is important in helping obstetrician–gynecologists develop such an understanding.

Theories of Aging

Aging often is equated with senescence and is defined as a constellation of changes in structure and function, generally beginning after sexual maturation. Two important concepts in understanding the normal aging process are homeostenosis and heterogeneity. *Homeostenosis* refers to the slow and progressive narrowing of physiologic reserve with increasing age and the accompanying decreased ability to withstand stress or injury. *Heterogeneity* refers to the wide range of differences in individuals who are at a point in the aging process when age no longer is closely correlated with functional capability. Similarly, different organ systems within an individual may age at different rates. Table 1 summarizes some age-related changes that occur in the various organ systems and their potential consequences.

There are several theories about the biologic basis of aging. Studies have estimated that between 70 and 7,000 genetic loci may be involved in the aging process, providing the basis for the theory that a series of programmed events occurs that leads to the changes during aging (2). A second theory, the free-radical theory of aging states that free radicals generated intracellularly are responsible for a host of oxidative alterations that are the root of cell alterations and cell death in aging aerobic organisms (3). A third theory states that somatic mutations occur during aging

Table 1. Age-Related Organ Systems Changes

Organ System	Age-Related Change	Potential Consequence
General	Increased body fat	Increased volume of distribution for fat-soluble drugs
	Decreased total body water	Decreased volume of distribution for water-soluble drugs
Ocular	Presbyopia	Decreased accommodation
	Lens opacification	Increased susceptibility to glare, need for increased illumination
	Macular degeneration	Blindness
Audio	Decreased high-frequency acuity	Difficulty discriminating words if background noise is present
Endocrine	Impaired glucose homeostasis	Increased glucose levels in response to acute illness, diabetes mellitus
	Decreased thyroxine production and clearance	Decreased thyroxine dose needed in hypothyroidism
	Increased antidiuretic hormone levels, decreased rennin and aldosterone levels	Decreased sodium levels, increased potassium levels
	Decreased vitamin D absorption and activation	Osteopenia
	Decreased estrogen and androgen levels	Osteoporosis, vaginal dryness, decreased libido
Respiratory	Decreased lung elasticity and increased chest wall stiffness	Ventilation and perfusion mismatch, decreased PO_2, dyspnea, hypoxia
Cardiovascular	Decreased arterial compliance and increased systolic blood pressure level, left ventricular hypertrophy	Hypotensive response to increased heart rate, volume depletion or loss of atrial contraction, syncope
	Decreased β-adrenergic responsiveness	Decreased cardiac output and heart rate response to stress, possible heart failure
	Decreased baroreceptor sensitivity and decreased sinoauricular node automaticity	Impaired blood pressure response to standing, volume depletion, possible heart block
Gastrointestinal	Decreased hepatic function	Delayed metabolism of some drugs
	Decreased gastric acidity	Decreased calcium absorption, vitamin B_{12} deficiency
	Decreased colonic mobility	Constipation, fecal impaction
	Decreased anorectal function	Fecal incontinence

(continued)

Table 1. Age-Related Organ Systems Changes *(continued)*

Organ System	Age-Related Change	Potential Consequence
Hematologic and immune	Possible decreased bone marrow reserve, impaired leukocytosis response to infection	Anemia
	Decreased T-cell function	False-negative test result of purified protein derivative test
	Increased autoantibodies	False-positive rheumatoid factor, antinuclear antibody, auto-immune disease test results
Renal	Decreased glomerular filtration rate	Impaired excretion of some drugs, increased serum creatinine concentration
	Decreased urine concentration and dilution	Delayed response to salt or fluid restriction or overload, nocturia
Genitourinary	Vaginal and urethral mucosal atrophy	Dyspareunia, bacteruria
Musculoskeletal	Decreased lean body mass, decreased lean muscle	Functional impairment
	Decreased bone density	Osteopenia, fractures
	Joint degeneration	Arthritis
Nervous	Neuronal degeneration and loss	Benign senescence, forgetful-ness, dementia, delirium
	Decreased brain catechol synthesis	Depression
	Decreased dopaminergic synthesis	Stiffer gait, Parkinson disease, poor fine muscle coordination
	Decreased righting reflexes	Increased body sway, falls
	Decreased stage 4 sleep	Early awakening, insomnia, fatigue

and that the body's ability to clear cells with these mutations or to produce reparative activity may decline (4). A fourth theory pertains to the nonenzymatic glycation of proteins. In this theory, it is proposed that glucose-mediated glycation of proteins is a major mediator of organ system aging and that glycation of DNA has a potential role in mutagenesis (5). A fifth theory, *clonal senescence,* is defined as the gradual attenuation of the growth of proliferating colonies of somatic cells culminating in populations of cells that are still viable but are unable to reproduce (6). Because the maintenance of integrity of many tissues in mammals depends on an orderly replacement of cells, it is possible that clonal senescence of certain critical cell types may contribute to the development of components of senescence, leading to tissue atrophy or inappropriate proliferation. It has been theorized that this consequence of clonal senescence may contribute to the precursors of age-related neoplasia.

Although the actual biologic basis of aging currently is unknown, it is clear that many ele9ments converge on cells and organs throughout life to create this basis. Some elements, such as the genetic makeup of the individual, may be difficult to modify, but other elements, such as diet, smoking, and other environmental exposures, are modifiable and may be capable of modulating changes associated with aging.

Frailty

Much research has lead to an understanding of the development of frailty, a commonly recognized clinical state, which has been assumed to be an inevitable consequence of advanced age. It is now evident that frailty is a clinical syndrome with identifiable risk factors, clinical presentations, and potential interventions. Frailty is characterized by diminished physiologic function of a number of organ systems, which leads to a decreased ability to withstand stress or injury, with consequent increased risk of morbidity and mortality. The key clinical features are unintentional weight loss of more than 10 lb during a period of 12 months, weakness, decreased muscle mass and strength, decreased walking speed, decreased physical activity, decreased endurance, and increased exhaustion during physical activity. The presence of three or more of these changes is considered indicative of frailty. Risk factors of frailty are increased age, female sex, presence of chronic disease, self-perceived poor health, and low educational and economic status. Biologic markers of frailty include increased levels of interleukin-6 and C-reactive protein, impaired immune system function, and neuroendocrine system dysfunction. Individuals with frailty are at increased risk of falls, susceptibility to acute illness, slow recovery from illness, hospitalization, disability, dependency, institutionalization, and death (7). A prominent feature is sarcopenia, defined as the age-associated decrease in skeletal muscle mass, with an associated decrease in strength and exercise tolerance.

Disability, which may both contribute to and be a consequence of frailty, becomes increasingly common with advancing age. *Disability* can be defined as impairment in the ability to carry out one or more functions necessary for independent living, such as impaired mobility, vision, hearing, speech, and motor strength. It can occur as a consequence of many acute and chronic diseases or as a consequence of frailty. Approximately 18% of women aged 65–74 years have disability, and the prevalence of disability increases to 31% in women aged 75–84 years and 53% in women older than 85 years. The presence and extent of disability can be documented by standardized assessment instruments, such as the Activities of Daily Living (8) and the Instrumental Activities of Daily Living (9) tools, which can be administered by office staff.

Screening

The annual visit is an ideal time to evaluate the health status of older patients, assess their functional ability, and screen for diseases so that acute and chronic conditions can be discovered early. The most important ingredients of the health maintenance visit are an accurate medical history and physical examination. The American College of Obstetricians and Gynecologists has published periodic assessments organized by age groups to assist physicians in obtaining important information during these visits (10). During a patient's first visit, a complete medical history should be obtained, including the reasons for the visit, present illnesses, all medical illnesses and surgical procedures that the patient has had, and all prescription and over-the-counter medications that the patient currently uses. A complete systems review also should be performed. It is wise to have the patient bring all medications she currently takes, including prescription medications, over-the-counter medications, alternative medications, and vitamin supplements, to her appointment. Any medication allergies or sensitivities should be noted. A family medical history should be obtained, including diseases and causes of death in all first-degree relatives, especially histories of heart disease, stroke, diabetes mellitus, dementia, and cancer. A social history should be taken, with a focus on the ability of the woman to care for herself and carry out her activities of daily living. Use of tobacco, alcohol, and illicit drugs should be noted, and the physician should recommend cessation or decrease of use as appropriate. Questions should be asked about exposure to secondhand smoke.

The patient's living situation should be noted, including other members of the patient's household, their relationship to the patient, and any evidence that the patient is experiencing intimidation or violence. It is appropriate to ask patients with chronic illness or of advanced age about health care proxies and advance directives. Histories of patients' occupations and hobbies should be noted and evaluated from the standpoint of safety. Additionally, a record of immunizations and a record of travel, particularly outside of the United States, should be obtained. If the visit is an interim visit, changes since the last visit should be noted. Much of this information can be obtained by trained office staff, using history forms, which provide a structured format for asking questions and for recording information.

A complete physical examination should be performed at each annual health maintenance visit. This examination may include an evaluation of vision and hearing. An assessment of cognitive function may be performed using one of the standard tools, such as the Folstein Mini Mental Status Examination, which can be administered by trained office staff if the patient or a family member mentions that the patient has difficulty remembering. A general neurologic examination also should be performed.

Cursory examination of the patient for visual and hearing impairments can be completed in the physician's office, but a patient aged 65 years or older with no risk factors should be evaluated every 1–2 years for evidence of glaucoma (increased anterior chamber pressure) and for the presence of cataracts (11). The ophthalmoscopic examination may help to detect cataracts in the lenses and retinal signs of macular degeneration and vascular disease. General testing of hearing also is useful and periodically should be recommended for older patients. If vision or hearing is found to be inadequate, corrective lenses or hearing aids can be recommended when appropriate. When necessary, patients can be referred for cataract surgery or other corrective eye procedures.

With the aid of a complete medical history and physical examination, it often is possible to detect diseases early and to order appropriate laboratory tests for specific diagnoses so that therapy may begin. Laboratory tests are useful, but many tests yield false-positive or false-negative results, depending on the sensitivity and specificity at which they are set. In addition to laboratory tests, risk factors are useful in identifying potential medical conditions that are common among older women (Box 1).

 Box 1. Risk Factors for Aging Women

Coronary artery disease
- ☑ Smoking
- ☑ Hypertension
- ☑ Diabetes mellitus
- ☑ Polycystic ovary syndrome
- ☑ Age older than 55 years
- ☑ Premature menopause
- ☑ Family history of premature coronary artery disease
- ☑ High-density lipoprotein level less than 40 mg/dL (negative risk factor high-density lipoprotein level greater than 60 mg/dL)
- ☑ Obesity
- ☑ Physical inactivity

Osteoporosis
- ☑ Family history of osteoporosis
- ☑ White or Asian race
- ☑ Hyperthyroidism
- ☑ Hyperparathyroidism
- ☑ Prolonged use of corticosteroids
- ☑ Smoking
- ☑ Alcohol abuse
- ☑ Early oophorectomy or premature menopause

(continued)

Box 1. Risk Factors for Aging Women *(continued)*

☑ History of lactose intolerance

☑ Sedentary lifestyle

☑ Immobilization

☑ Small lean body habitus

☑ Low calcium, vitamin D, or dairy product intake

Breast cancer

☑ Age

☑ Family history of breast cancer or other types of cancer

☑ Heavy radiation exposure

☑ History of breast cancer

☑ Carcinoma in situ of the breast found on biopsy

☑ Atypical hyperplasia

☑ History of multiple breast biopsies

Ovarian cancer

☑ Age

☑ Family history

☑ New onset of bloating, abdominal discomfort, and bowel symptoms

Colorectal cancer

☑ Age

☑ First-degree relatives with colon cancer

☑ History of colorectal cancer, breast cancer, endometrial cancer, or ovarian cancer

☑ History of adenomatous polyps

☑ Ulcerative colitis

(continued)

Box 1. Risk Factors for Aging Women
(continued)

Melanoma

☑ Fair skin and hair color

☑ History of sun exposure over time or severe sunburn

☑ Family history of melanoma

☑ Large congenital nevi

☑ Presence of pigmented lesions meeting the criteria for dysplastic nevi
—Macular and papular components
—Irregular borders
—Variegated pigmentation within the same lesion
—Diameter of 5–12 mm

Coronary Artery Disease

Coronary artery disease is a major health risk in women. Each year, 2.5 million women are hospitalized in the United States because of cardiovascular disease, and in 2004, more than 330,000 women aged 65 years and older died of heart disease (1). Thus, it is important for health care providers to identify risk factors wherever possible by treating hypertension and diabetes mellitus and encouraging healthy practices, such as smoking cessation, good nutrition, and regular exercise.

The National Cholesterol Education Program recommends that all adults undergo a fasting lipoprotein profile every 5 years (12). Hypercholesteremia should be addressed medically whenever possible. A low-fat, low-calorie diet should be recommended for all patients with low-density lipoprotein (LDL) values of 130 mg/dL or greater and two or more of the previously mentioned risk factors and for patients with LDL levels of 160 mg/dL or greater even if they have no risk factors. Drug therapy should be started in postmenopausal women if their LDL levels are

160 mg/dL or greater and they have two or more risk factors or if their LDL levels are 190 mg/dL or greater and they have no risk factors. In addition, if coronary artery disease has been diagnosed, diet therapy should be started if the LDL level is 100 mg/dL or greater, and drug therapy should be started if the LDL level is 130 mg/dL or greater (12).

Stroke

Cerebrovascular disease is the third leading cause of death in the United States after heart disease and cancer (1). Women should be screened for risk factors for stroke, which include hypertension, dyslipidemia, diabetes mellitus, smoking, and use of hormone therapy.

Hypertension

The Seventh Report of the Joint National Committee on Prevention, Detection, Evaluation, and Treatment of High Blood Pressure includes a revised blood pressure classification (13) (Table 2). Generally, individuals with mild hypertension can be treated with diet and exercise regimens (14), which should be used before drug therapy is considered. Drug therapy should be used for patients with stage 1 and stage 2 hypertension (13). Cessation of smoking and reduction of blood pressure levels of participants in the Systolic Hypertension in the Elderly Program resulted in 36% fewer fatal and nonfatal strokes and 27% fewer fatal and nonfatal myocardial infarctions in treated individuals compared with the control group (15). These benefits were noted in all groups regardless of age, race, sex, or blood pressure subgroup.

Table 2. Classification of Blood Pressure for Adults

Classification	Systolic (mm Hg)	Diastolic (mm Hg)
Normal	Less than 120	And less than 80
Prehypertension	120–139	Or 80–89
Stage 1 hypertension	140–159	Or 90–99
Stage 2 hypertension	160 or greater	Or 100 or greater

Modified from National Heart, Lung, and Blood Institute. National High Blood Pressure Education Program. The seventh report of the Joint National Committee on Prevention, Detection, Evaluation, and Treatment of High Blood Pressure. Bethesda (MD): NHLBI; 2003.

Diabetes Mellitus

Diabetes mellitus is a group of diseases characterized by the inability to process glucose properly. Type 1 diabetes mellitus occurs because of the destruction of pancreatic islet cells. Although it usually occurs in childhood, it may occur any time in life. Type 2 diabetes mellitus is the predominant type seen in older individuals. It is associated with impairment of insulin release and resistance to insulin action. The prevalence of diabetes mellitus among individuals aged 60 years or older in the United States was 23.1% in 2007 (16). Long-term complications include cardiovascular disease, renal failure, neuropathy, and blindness.

Many authorities recommend that patients at high risk for type 2 diabetes mellitus, such as obese individuals, individuals with family histories of diabetes mellitus, and women who have had gestational diabetes mellitus be screened. The American College of Obstetricians and Gynecologists recommends the administration of a fasting glucose test every 3 years for women older than 45 years (10). For patients with glucose intolerance (a fasting glucose level of 106–125 mg/dL), diet therapy and weight loss can be useful. An elevated fasting glucose level (a fasting glucose level greater than or equal to 126 mg/dL) or 2-hour postprandial glucose level greater than 200 mg/dL is indicative of individuals with overt diabetes mellitus.

Thyroid Disease

Both hypothyroidism and subclinical hypothyroidism are more common in older individuals. Signs and symptoms associated with this condition in older women (Box 2) may differ from those in younger women. Individuals with hypothyroidism often have increased body mass indexes (BMIs) and may have elevated cholesterol levels. The prevalence of hypothyroidism in otherwise healthy individuals is approximately 5%. *Subclinical hypothyroidism,* defined as serum thyrotropin levels greater than normal in the presence of normal levels of serum thyroxine, free thyroxine, triiodothyronine, and free triiodothyronine, occurs in approximately 15% of women older than 65 years (17). Thyrotropin level measurement is a good assessment tool. The American Thyroid Association recommends that all adults aged 35 years or older be screened by measurement of serum thyrotropin levels, with repeated screening every

> ## Box 2. Signs and Symptoms of Hypothyroidism in Older Women
>
> - Fatigue
> - Lethargy
> - Constipation
> - Memory impairment
> - Depression
> - Feeling of coldness and cold intolerance
> - Dry skin
> - Thinning of scalp hair
> - Delayed relaxation phase of reflexes

5 years; patients with risk factors for thyroid dysfunction may need to be screened more often (18). Individuals with elevated cholesterol levels or symptoms of hypothyroidism should be screened, and other individuals should probably be screened periodically. In older women, increased cholesterol levels that may be associated with subclinical hypothyroidism may increase patients' risk of coronary artery disease and peripheral vascular disease.

Hyperthyroidism is less common in older women, but does occur. Signs and symptoms that may be seen in this condition are shown in Box 3. Older individuals also may present with atrial fibrillation or congestive heart failure; therefore, individuals with these symptoms should be screened (19, 20). *Subclinical hyperthyroidism*, defined as suppressed serum thyrotropin levels and normal levels of serum thyroxine, free thyroxine, triiodothyronine, and free triiodothyronine, often is associated with accelerated osteoporosis, increased risk of atrial fibrillation, and an overall increased risk of death and may develop in women with long-standing nodular goiter who were previously euthyroid.

Anemia

Anemia is common in older women (21, 22). Iron-deficiency anemia, vitamin B_{12} deficiency, and folate deficiency all occur in this pop-

---

Box 3. Signs and Symptoms of Hyperthyroidism in Older Women

- Easy fatigue and decreased energy
- Weight loss
- Muscle weakness
- Palpitations
- Increased sweating
- Heat intolerance
- Increased frequency of bowel movements
- Rapid pulse
- Atrial fibrillation
- Increased systolic blood pressure
- Lid lag (exophthalmos is rare)
- Osteopenia and osteoporosis

---

ulation. Iron-deficiency anemia may be associated with blood loss, such as loss from a gastrointestinal source. Although there is some controversy about performing a complete blood count annually, there is agreement that a hematocrit measurement should be obtained. If anemia is found, the type should be defined and its causality determined and treated.

Osteoporosis

Osteoporosis occurs because of increased bone resorption with reduced bone formation. This reduction leads to decreased bone density and increased likelihood of vertebral, hip, and long bone fracture (23). It generally is a slow process, beginning in the fourth decade of life, and is accelerated by several risk factors. The American College of Obstetricians and Gynecologists recommends bone mineral density testing in all postmenopausal women aged 65 years or older (24). Bone mineral density testing may be recommended for postmenopausal women younger than 65 years who have one or more risk factors for osteoporosis (24).

Bone density assessments should be repeated every 1–2 years in women with risk factors for osteoporosis. Hormone therapy reduces the risk of osteoporosis but does not stop the process completely. Hormone therapy should not be initiated solely for reducing the risk of osteoporosis because the risk of this therapy may outweigh the benefits. The use of other medications, such as selective estrogen receptor modulators (ie, raloxifene) and bisphosphonates, such as alendronate and risedronate, is effective. The use of statins has been reported to increase bone density and may be useful in treating osteopenia and osteoporosis in patients who are already taking this medication for lipid management; however, these drugs are not yet accepted as initial therapies for osteoporosis.

Cancer

Ideally, it is desirable to detect cancer in either the precancerous or early invasive stage. Early detection of cervical cancer is possible with the use of cervical cytology tests, and early detection of breast cancer is possible with the use of mammography. It is more difficult to detect lung cancer and ovarian cancer, which may be quite advanced before the patient has symptoms. Colorectal cancer and endometrial cancer may be detected relatively early because of their tendency to cause bleeding. Any postmenopausal vaginal bleeding and either occult or overt rectal bleeding should be investigated immediately. Many types of cancer are more common in older individuals, and cancer is the second leading cause of death in older individuals. The incidence of lung cancer in women has increased dramatically in the past 50 years, probably because of an increased number of women who smoke (25, 26). In 2008, it was estimated that 71,030 women in the United States would die from lung cancer and 40,480 women would die from breast cancer even though the incidence of breast cancer is much greater (182,460 new cases of breast cancer estimated in 2008 compared with 100,330 new cases of lung cancer) (27).

Routine screening for cervical cancer by cervical cytology testing should be performed throughout a woman's lifetime. In women aged 65 years or older, the American College of Obstetricians and Gynecologists recommends cervical cytology tests every 2–3 years after 3 consecutive negative test results in women with no history of cervical intraepithelial neoplasia 2 or 3, immunosuppression, human immunodeficiency virus (HIV) infection, or diethylstilbestrol exposure in utero (28). There is no consensus of when annual cervical cytology tests can be discontinued. The American Cancer Society recommends that cervical cytology tests can be discontinued at age 70 years in women with low risk of cervical cancer (29), whereas the U.S. Preventive Services Task Force recommends that cervical cytology tests can be discontinued at age 65 years in women with low risk (30).

Age is definitely a risk factor for breast cancer, with approximately a 2% incidence at age 50 years and a 12% incidence at age 90 years (31, 32). Minor risk factors include nulliparity, late first pregnancy, early menarche, and late menopause. There are several other possible risk factors, including prolonged hormone therapy, high-fat diet, obesity, moderate-to-heavy alcohol use, and sedentary lifestyle. The known risk factors account for only one half of cases of breast cancer, and all women should be screened as recommended. The American Cancer Society recommends yearly mammography beginning at age 40 years. The American College of Obstetricians and Gynecologists recommends mammography every 1–2 years beginning at age 40 years and continued annually after age 50 years throughout a woman's lifetime (29, 33).

Ovarian cancer is a common and often lethal disease. There are no screening tests with good sensitivity or specificity that allow for the detection of this disease at an early stage. Studies using pelvic ultrasonography and the measurement of tumor markers such as CA 125 have not been proved effective. When the disease becomes clinically detectable, it usually is in an advanced stage with a poor prognosis. Classically, it has been considered a silent cancer in its early stages, but results of recent research suggest that frequent symptoms of bloating and abdominal discomfort and bowel symptoms in patients who have not had previous conditions related to these symptoms might suggest the development of ovarian cancer, and these patients should receive further evaluation. Although the relationship of these symptoms to the disease may be present, it has yet to be seen whether laboratory testing in the presence of these symptoms leads to an earlier diagnosis or positively affects the cure rate (34).

In 2008, it was estimated that 71,560 women in the United States would develop colorectal cancer (27). Individuals at highest risk are those who have two or more first-degree relatives with colorectal cancer, family cancer syndromes, or family histories of polyposis coli. Most colon cancers arise from adenomatous polyps in the distal colon and may be seen on endoscopic examination (35). Not all polyps become cancer, and the degeneration to cancer generally takes 5–10 years. The American College of Obstetricians and Gynecologists recommends screening women at average risk of colorectal cancer beginning at age 50 years (more specific recommendations are given for women at high risk) (36). The preferred method of screening is colonoscopy. Women who have positive fecal occult blood test results should undergo colonoscopy. Individuals in high-risk groups may be tested more frequently with colonoscopy.

The risk of skin cancer increases with age. An annual full-skin examination is recommended for individuals older than 50 years to detect evidence of squamous cell cancer, basal cell cancer, and melanoma. These types of cancer are commonly found in areas that are exposed to the sun (ie, the head and neck) (37). Squamous cell cancer arises from actinic keratosis. When keratotic lesions are found, they may be destroyed with liquid nitrogen. Squamous cell tumors or basal cell tumors should be removed surgically.

Vulvar Lesions

Older women may have a variety of benign and malignant vulvar conditions that may present with itching, pigmentation change, or lesions. The vulva should be inspected carefully, and areas of recent pigmentation, excoriation, white (keratotic) epithelium, or lesion should undergo biopsy. Lichen sclerosus, epithelial hyperplasia, Paget disease, vulvar carcinoma, and melanoma are all seen in this age group.

Special Issues

As patients age, they become more vulnerable to certain conditions. Obstetrician–gynecologists should be aware of the special issues that affect their older patients.

Abuse and Violence

Older women are vulnerable to domestic abuse and violence. The abuse may be physical, including sexual assault; emotional; psychologic; or financial. Abuse also includes neglect and abandonment. Abused women older than 75 years often are physically or cognitively impaired and generally are widowed and living with relatives. The abuser often is an adult child or grandchild within the family but may be any other household member.

Physicians caring for older patients should be aware of signs and symptoms of domestic abuse. Abused women may have frequent somatic symptoms, such as headaches; digestive disorders; or chest, back, or pelvic pain. Mental health symptoms that may be present include feelings of inadequacy, self-blame, evidence of substance or alcohol abuse, and a history of suicide attempts (38). In addition, physical evidence, such as bruises, scratches, or burns, often are noted. If these injuries are observed, the patient should be asked how she received them. It is appropriate to ask older women if anyone in their household or among their acquaintances has injured them, threatened to injure them, or made other threats or intimidated them in any way. Widowed women living with family members are particularly susceptible and should be asked these questions routinely (39).

All 50 states have passed legislation to help protect older individuals from domestic violence and neglect. Most states have mandatory reporting laws. Older women who are found to have experienced abuse or intimidation should be counseled about their rights, which center on the fact that they have the right to not be intimidated or abused. Social service agencies, the police, and other legal agencies may be consulted, with the permission of the patient, to either remove the perpetrator from the home or to find a safe haven for the patient. Physicians can help these patients by identifying abusive situations and helping patients identify their options.

Depression

It has been shown that 50–60% of patient visits to primary care physicians are for problems that have a behavioral or emotional component, and 25% of the patients visiting primary care physicians have psychiatric disorders (40). Women have a much greater lifetime risk of depression than men (41).

Depression is common in older women and may be associated with bereavement, disappointment, or other types of loss. It may be transient and frequently requires no therapy. Mild antidepressive agents may be helpful over the short term.

Major depression, however, is a larger problem. Women with depression may appear apathetic, tired, sad, and disinterested. They often speak slowly, have difficulty concentrating, and answer questions after several seconds of delay. In some older patients, depression can mimic dementia. Many times, in patients with depression, the condition is not diagnosed by primary care physicians because health care providers often focus on symptoms rather than on the whole patient, and patients may disguise their symptoms. The American Psychiatric Association has developed criteria for diagnosing a major depressive episode that include depressed mood; diminished interest or pleasure; weight loss or appetite change; insomnia or hypersomnia; psychomotor agitation or retardation; fatigue or loss of energy; feelings of worthlessness or guilt; difficulty thinking, concentrating, or making decisions; and recurring thoughts of death or suicide (42).

If a patient is depressed, it is important to determine if she is suicidal. It is appropriate to ask her directly, "Have you thought of injuring yourself or taking your life?" If the answer is yes, it is important to ascertain if she has taken steps to carry this out. Women who entertain thoughts of suicide or are planning to commit suicide require acute management and should be immediately referred to a mental health specialist.

Women who are not suicidal but have evidence of depression may be considered for treatment with three basic models: 1) the medication model, 2) the psychologic treatment model, and 3) the social model. Often, a combination of these three models is necessary for the individual patient.

MEDICATION MODEL

The medication model involves the use of antidepressant drugs. There are two classes of these drugs: 1) the selective serotonin uptake inhibitors, such as fluoxetine, sertraline, paroxetine, and

serotonin norepinephrine reuptake inhibitors and 2) tricyclic medications, such as amitriptyline, doxepin, and imipramine; however this latter group often yields a poor response in older
women. There also are several new medications that are being
introduced. Antidepressant medications require up to 1 month of
use to be effective; instant improvement usually is caused by a
placebo effect and will not necessarily continue. Patients should
be cautioned that they will not feel better for up to 1 month and
that the dose may require adjustment. As with any medication,
there can be side effects. Tricyclics usually have an anticholinergic effect that may cause dryness in the mouth, urinary retention,
constipation, blurred vision, and, at times, delirium in older
patients, making the use of these drugs in this age group less
desirable. Occasionally, blood pressure levels will decrease sub-
stantially, leading to a tendency for the patient to faint when she
arises at night. Selective serotonin reuptake inhibitors may cause
a decrease in appetite and sexual desire (43) but usually are more
effective in this age group.

PSYCHOLOGIC TREATMENT MODEL

The psychologic treatment model consists of either psychotherapy
or self-help therapy. It is aimed at solving social problems that
are contributing to the depression. These may be interpersonal
relationships, problems with trust and coping, or difficulty solving problems. Patients also may have a parental history of psychologic disorders, history of alcohol abuse, personality disorders,
or history of emotional, physical, or sexual abuse (43).

SOCIAL MODEL

The final model is the social model, which integrates the assis-
tance and resources of social service agencies and social workers.
This model is most helpful in treating depression caused by
domestic violence, severe financial difficulty, social isolation,
bereavement, or decrease in functional abilities.

Dementia

Dementia, which involves the destruction of brain cells caused by
organic brain damage, is common in older women. It is defined
as an acquired, chronic, progressive, irreversible impairment in

cognition. It affects multiple domains of cognition, including memory, speech, arithmetic ability, spatial–temporal orientation, personality, and judgment.

Approximately 3–5% of individuals will have dementia by age 65 years. More than 20% of individuals will experience severe dementia by the age of 80 years, and as many as 50% will be affected by the age of 90 years (44). With dementia, there is impairment of both short-term and long-term memory, abstract thinking, and the ability to logically consider and solve problems. Women who experience dementia may have difficulty putting thoughts into words and may even have difficulty speaking.

Older individuals often have symptoms of memory impairment; however, it is important to understand that these symptoms do not always indicate the presence of dementia. Some individuals who are concerned about memory function will have age-associated memory impairment, also known as benign senescent forgetfulness. Psychometric testing in individuals with this condition will produce normal results for age, and these patients can be assured that their condition probably will not progress to dementia. More important is the detection of mild cognitive impairment. Individuals with mild cognitive impairment have symptoms of impaired memory and objective changes in memory function on testing, but they do not have other cognitive impairments or impairment in carrying out daily activities. It is essential that these individuals be evaluated periodically because approximately 15% will show progression to overt dementia in 1 year and by 5 years 50% will have dementia.

Dementia is caused by a number of conditions that result in the destruction of neurons (Box 4). The most common causes of dementia are Alzheimer disease; cerebrovascular disease, including stroke and multiple lacunar infarcts; Parkinson disease; Lewy bodies; frontotemporal dementia; and normal pressure hydrocephalus. Regardless of the cause, the damage to the brain is irreversible.

Patients with some forms of dementia may experience motor function impairment, causing gait difficulty or difficulty performing tasks. Along with these changes, there are almost always personality changes (43). When dementia is suspected, the patient should be referred to a geriatric specialist or a neurologist who has the ability to specifically diagnose the condition and offer therapy.

Box 4. Causes of Dementia and Delirium

Dementia

- Alzheimer disease
- Multiple vascular infarcts
- Lewy bodies
- Parkinson disease
- Frontal lobe dementia
- Advanced HIV infection
- Chronic alcoholism
- Normal pressure hydrocephalus
- Pick disease
- Creutzfeldt–Jakob disease

Delirium

- Infection (urinary tract, respiratory system)
- Exposure to external toxins and drugs
- Electrolyte imbalance, hypercalcemia, hyponatremia
- Anemia, hypoxia (poor oxygenation)
- Metabolic problems, hypothyroidism, hyperpara-thyroidism
- Hypoglycemia
- Central nervous system infections

Delirium

Delirium is an organic brain disorder caused by altered brain physiology. As such, it is reversible if the underlying cause can be identified and corrected. It is commonly seen in older patients when the brain undergoes a global disruption of metabolic equilibrium, which may be caused by a variety of conditions. The diagnostic criteria for delirium include disturbance of consciousness and change in cognition, developing over a short period of time, and evidence from the history, physical examination, or laboratory results that the disturbance is caused by the direct physiologic consequences of a general medical condition (42).

Delirium generally begins with a sudden onset of mental status change, usually marked by disorientation, confusion, inability to remember new information, and varying levels of consciousness (43). These symptoms may vary over hours from near-normal mental status to substantial impairment of orientation. The patient may appear sleepy, hallucinate, or lose sense of time. Delirium frequently occurs postoperatively in older women who have had surgical procedures and may be caused by a transient lack of oxygen, an imbalance of fluids or electrolytes, the use of drugs with central nervous system activity (analgesics), infections, a decreased ability of the body to nourish brain cells (such as with hypoglycemia), or other metabolic disorders related to the anesthetic or operation itself. It also may occur in patients who are using certain drugs that cannot be promptly cleared from the body. One such drug is diazepam, the use of which should be avoided by older women. Treatment of delirium usually involves support of the patient and the removal of its cause. In most cases, recognition is the most important factor in beginning therapy. However, susceptibility to delirium in older women may be an indication of dementia or physiologic brittleness and may have severe prognostic implications, with respect to longevity. In one study, 13% of patients hospitalized after the age of 70 years developed delirium, which led to higher health care costs that rivaled falls and diabetes mellitus, with a shorter survival time (45).

CASE NO. 1. A frail 71-year-old patient with recurrent breast cancer is frightened about impending death and is in moderate pain from bone metastases that is partially controlled with the use of oral analgesia. Her physician prescribed diazepam, 10 mg, twice daily, for her anxiety. Her condition improved during the first week; however, she gradually developed hallucinations and loss of perception of time and place. She was hospitalized for observation of possible psychosis. It became evident that she was experiencing delirium. The use of diazepam was discontinued, and her delirium cleared within 3 days.

Older, frail patients metabolize many medications, including
diazepam, slowly. Because of this, many physicians will not prescribe diazepam for use in older adults. Because the patient experienced anxiety and agitation before beginning the medication,
her delirium was initially misdiagnosed as a psychotic reaction.

Falls

Falls in older women can have serious health consequences,
including death. In 2005, more than 15,800 individuals aged 65
years and older died, and at least 1.8 million individuals were
injured as a result of falls. In individuals aged 65 years and older,
falls are the leading cause of injury, disability, and deaths caused
by injuries (46). The risk factors for falls include older age, muscle
weakness, functional limitations, use of certain medications or
combinations of medications, disorders that can affect balance,
and a history of falls. Recurrent falls often are a marker for underlying disease or impaired physiologic function and are associated
with a high risk of severe morbidity and death. Many women
with frequent falls will develop "fear of falling" and markedly
limit their activities, including excursions outside the home, with
resultant social isolation and decreased mobility, which further
increases the risk for falling.

Soft tissue injuries are a common consequence of falls among
older women. Hip fracture is the most common serious injury
caused by falling, and approximately 76% of all hip fractures
occur in women (47). In 2004, more than 320,000 individuals
were hospitalized with hip fractures. The rate of hip fracture is
expected to increase as the population of older individuals
increases.

At the annual examination, physicians should evaluate their
older patients' risk factors for falling. They should examine their
patients' gait and balance by observing them sitting and standing
from a chair and walking (48). Physicians also should ask their
patients if they have experienced any falls. If they have, physicians should ask about the circumstances so they can determine
any factors that may have contributed to the fall. The National
Institute on Aging has created a web page with recommendations
for patients to prevent falls (see Resources). In addition to these
recommendations, older women can be advised to remove throw

rugs and other tripping hazards from walkways, use nonskid mats in bathtubs and showers, use handrails in bathrooms and on stairs, and keep rooms well lit. Multifactorial assessments and targeted interventions for preventing falls have been shown to prevent falls in older individuals (49).

Pelvic Support Problems

When a physician performs a pelvic examination on an older woman, pelvic support problems become obvious. At this point, it is important to determine if the patient is symptomatic because of the relaxation of pelvic supports. If defects are found and the patient is symptomatic, the physician must determine which supports are damaged and if surgical intervention or nonsurgical treatment with a pessary and possibly hormone therapy would be of use. The choice of therapy depends on the degree of the patient's symptoms, the patient's ability to withstand surgical intervention, and her ability to use other interventions, such as a pessary. This should be determined on an individual basis.

Urinary Incontinence

Urinary incontinence is common in older women. Between 5% and 15% of older women living in their own homes have some form of urinary incontinence (50). Furthermore, up to 40% of women older than 70 years who are hospitalized and as many as 40–60% of women in nursing homes are incontinent of urine (51, 52). Social embarrassment associated with incontinence may be so great that it may cause women to limit social contact outside the home and perhaps lose employment opportunities. Women also may be too embarrassed to tell their physicians they experience urinary incontinence. Therefore, physicians should ask patients if they ever experience urinary incontinence. In patients who do experience urinary incontinence, physicians should determine how often and under what circumstances it occurs and if incontinence pads or protective garments are routinely used. In addition, patients should be asked if any medical or surgical interventions have been attempted and the degree of success.

Urinary incontinence is a complicated issue, involving interaction of patients' neurologic states, mental statuses, and anatomic and hormonal balances. In many cases, medication use may cause urinary incontinence. Physicians should consider these factors when determining the cause of urinary incontinence.

Urinary continence occurs because the urethra contracts and the bladder relaxes, allowing urine to be stored and not passed. Both the urethra and the bladder are under the control of the autonomic nervous system, and urinary continence is controlled by the sympathetic nervous system through the neurotransmitter norepinephrine. Because the urethra and lower bladder neck have several α-receptors, their stimulation causes muscle contraction. The bladder only has β-receptors, so their stimulation by norepinephrine causes relaxation. Stimulation of the sympathetic nervous system supports urinary continence. However, the parasympathetic nervous system is responsible for micturition. Through the parasympathetic neurotransmitter acetylcholine, bladder musculature will contract, and the upper urethral musculature will relax. Medications that affect either of these neurotransmitters or receptor sites may interfere with continence or the ability to void. Table 3 provides examples of possible side effects of medications on the lower urinary tract.

The physician's primary objective with respect to urinary incontinence is to identify the condition in the patient, assess whether it is a concern for her, and, if it is, adequately evaluate her and offer treatment specific to her particular condition. In older women, detrusor hyperreflexia and urge urinary incontinence are common, especially in nursing home patients, and should be considered as causes of urinary incontinence during the evaluation of these patients.

CASE NO. 2. A 91-year-old patient who lives in a nursing home is referred because her nurses state that she is incontinent and is difficult to care for. She has moderately advanced Alzheimer disease. The patient is referred because the nurses hope that her incontinence can be addressed.

At examination, the patient has total prolapse of her vagina, cervix, and uterus, and there are several ulcers on her vagina. She clearly is incontinent. The family member and nurse who accompanied her indicate that they support correction of her pelvic prolapse and an effort to address her incontinence even though they have been told that this might be difficult because the primary contributing factor might not be an anatomic disorder or detrusor hyperreflexia.

The patient was given vaginal estrogen cream and fitted for a pessary (this required several attempts). During a 3-month period, the ulcers healed, and the vaginal epithelium appeared healthy. After medical consultation, colpocleisis (LeFort procedure) and Kelly plication of the bladder neck was performed. A local anesthesia was used.

The patient tolerated the procedure well and, although she still experienced nocturia, the nursing home nurses believed that her incontinence was improved and that she was less difficult to care for because of her reduced prolapse. Although it was impossible to completely correct this patient's incontinence, the improvement in her health and well-being was beneficial to her and her caregivers.

Table 3. Possible Side Effects of Medication on the Lower Urinary Tract

Medication	Side Effects	Consequence
Diuretics	Polyuria, nocturia	Urgency, frequency
Antihypertensives (reserpine, methyldopa)	Incontinence	Depleted catecholamines
Calcium channel blockers	Urinary retention and overflow incontinence	Increased bladder storage (relaxes smooth muscle)
Dopaminergic agents (bromocriptine, levodopa)	Bladder neck obstruction	Increased urethral resistance and decreased detrusor contractions
Cholinergic agonists (digitalis)	Decreased bladder capacity and increased intravesical pressure	Increased bladder wall tension
Anticholinergic agents (antihistamines, antidepressants, antipsychotics, opiates, antispasmodics, antiparkinsonian drugs, β-adrenergic agonists)	Decreased detrusor activity	Urinary retention
Xanthines (caffeine)	Incontinence	Decreased urethral pressure

Anal Incontinence

Many elderly women also are incontinent of flatus or stool. Patients may be too embarrassed to mention symptoms of this condition to their physicians and should be asked about such symptoms. Anatomic or neurologic damage may be the cause of this condition. Occasionally, stool impaction may be the cause. If symptoms of anal incontinence are present and worrisome to a patient, the symptoms should be evaluated.

Sexuality

With advancing age, most women experience a decrease in sexual function and satisfaction. Sexuality also may be influenced by a woman's health, her partner's health, medication use, and physiologic state as well as individual importance placed on sexual activity as a source of comfort and gratification.

In one study of more than 4,000 adults older than 50 years, most individuals stated that they were still sexually active (53). Individuals who were sexually active reported happier marriages and relationships than did sexually inactive individuals of the same age. Generally, older women showed a more marked reduction than men in the desire to remain sexually active. Masturbation levels remained stable in women, but decreased in men, with age. Other studies have shown a reduction in orgasmic response in older women. In one study, 49% of the women reported a decrease in sexual activity after menopause, 38% reported no change, and 15% reported an increase in sexual interest (54). Older women and men often report an increased interest in caressing and mutual masturbation, but a decreased interest in intercourse.

The sexual performance of older women often is related to the ability of their partners, and, therefore, relates as much to the health and vigor of the partner as to the health and vigor of the woman herself. Women who perceive their marriages to be good generally have greater satisfaction in their sexual relationships (55). Women who experience depression frequently note a decrease in sexual satisfaction.

After menopause, estrogen, progesterone, and testosterone levels are decreased. The thickness and elasticity of the vagina and urinary tract may be decreased, as is the amount of vaginal lubrication, even in women receiving hormone therapy. Acidity of the vagina usually decreases after menopause, and these women may be more susceptible to vaginal irritation and low-grade infections.

There often is an increase in the amount of time necessary for sexual arousal and a decrease in the number and intensity of orgasmic contractions after menopause (56). Loss of elasticity and smoothness of facial and body skin may be perceived as a loss of attractiveness and may contribute to a decrease in sexual interest in one or both members of the couple. Medication use may affect many aspects of sexual response, and psychosocial factors may influence a couple's desire for sexual activity. Some cultural stereotypes of older individuals include a perception that they may be desexualized or unattractive, so older women may believe their sexual desires are abnormal. Because women outlive men, older women may have fewer opportunities for relationships. In addition, older women may experience losses that may lead to a grief reaction, and this may limit the amount of emotional energy available for sexual activity.

With a lack of estrogen, genital appearance may change, including thinning and dryness of the vaginal epithelium, decrease of fullness of the clitoris and labia, and a reduction in pubic hair. The vagina may shrink in length and become narrow in diameter. If intercourse is not practiced for a long time, the vagina may actually close with adhesions and atrophy. As atrophy develops in the vaginal tissue, women are more susceptible to vaginal infection, vaginal tears, and other irritations. These factors may cause a woman to avoid intercourse.

Because sexual function is influenced by the autonomic nervous system, use of medications that affect the autonomic nervous system may affect sexual desire or orgasm. The parasympathetic nervous system, via the neurotransmitter acetylcholine, is responsible for arousal. Thus, use of medications that interfere with acetylcholine will frequently decrease sexual desire. Women affected by this often state that when they attempt sexual relations, they become aroused after a period of time and have normal orgasm. However, use of medications that interfere with the sympathetic nervous system by interfering with the neurotransmitter norepinephrine may block orgasm. Women affected by this circumstance may note normal arousal, but may not be able to attain a normal degree of orgasmic function or any orgasm at all. Likewise, men also may be influenced by medications that affect the autonomic nervous system and may experience impotence or difficulty maintaining an erection. It is appropriate to discuss sexual function with patients and, if it appears that medication may be interfering with normal function, it may be possible to adjust medications to alleviate this problem.

It is extremely important to obtain a detailed medical history from each patient to determine if the patient is sexually active, if the patient wishes to be sexually active, and if the patient has a partner who is capable of sexual activity. If the patient has problems in this area, the physician should determine the cause of these problems and rectify them if possible. Results of research have shown an increase in sexual interest with the presence of a new partner. This information is important for the physician to keep in mind when treating a divorced or widowed patient.

A few types of sexual dysfunction may occur in older women. One such disorder is vaginismus. This condition generally is a result of a painful vaginal experience, ranging from irritation caused by infection, scarring after surgery, or sexual assault. The problem should be viewed as a defensive reaction and, when the cause has been removed, such as treating an infection, dilating or cutting adhesions, or dealing with the assault on a psychosocial basis, the patient may be offered desensitizing exercises. Generally, these consist of digital dilation of the vagina, first by the patient, and then by her partner, in a safe situation over time without attempting intercourse. When the levator ani muscles, which have been in spasm, are taught to relax, intercourse may be attempted. Occasionally, vaginal dilators may be used in a progressive manner for this purpose. Treating vaginismus with desensitizing exercises is not difficult and is almost always successful if the cause has been removed (57).

Women who experience anorgasmia or difficulty in achieving orgasm may be helped by learning masturbatory techniques. These can be taught to or shared with their partners. An increase in stimulation, especially in the area of the clitoris, often is necessary to bring about orgasm in some older women. Occasionally, a vibrator may be used for stimulation during coitus to help with orgasm (57).

Dyspareunia may lead to vaginismus, but, because of the painful experience, it also may limit the amount of coital activity that the patient attempts. In each case, a careful evaluation and investigation of the cause should be performed, and, where possible, the problem should be alleviated.

Physicians often are reluctant to address issues of a sexual nature with their patients, but patients need to know that sexuality is a normal psychosocial activity, which can and should be enjoyed by older individuals. A caring physician who asks the correct questions may be in a position to perform an important and appreciated service to older women by helping them and their partners continue this normal function.

> **CASE NO. 3.** A 61-year-old woman visits the office for her annual examination and is asked about her sexual function. She states that she and her husband no longer have intercourse and she fears he is having an affair. For the past 6 months, he has demonstrated no sexual interest in her. On further questioning, she states that hypertension had been diagnosed in her husband 6 months earlier and he had started taking β-blockers. Neither she nor her husband had considered that his lack of sexual desire could be caused by the use of this medication.

Sexual dysfunction in men frequently is caused by medication use, and couples rarely discuss this concern. In this case, the patient's husband simply believed that his sexual interest had decreased, and the patient believed that her husband was no longer interested in her sexually. This is a common misinterpretation in such situations. Beta-blockers frequently cause erectile dysfunction. Calcium channel blockers also may cause erectile dysfunction, but they do so less frequently. The patient's husband discussed the matter with his internist who changed his medication to a calcium channel blocker, and his sexual interest improved. In this case, the erectile dysfunction ended when the medication was changed.

Grief and Loss

Everyone experiences loss. Loss may include the end of a relationship, the loss of a friend or relative by separation or death, the inability to conceive, miscarriage, the death of a child, or the loss of a job. For older individuals, losses may tend to accumulate, including the ability to participate in sports and other activities and the loss of pets. Pet loss in some older individuals may cause a severe reaction because older individuals may be limited in their contact with others (58).

Any loss may produce a grief reaction, which usually is accompanied by both physical and emotional symptoms. The grief reaction is described as a tightening of the throat and chest, a choking sensation, shortness of breath, frequent sighing, an empty feeling in the abdomen, muscle weakness, a feeling of tension and mental pain, and guilt (59). Most of these symptoms usually occur acutely after a loss. They may last for as long as 6–24 months, depending on the ability of the individual to replace the loss. Cultural variations exist and may influence the way in which an individual grieves.

The death of a child is probably the most severe loss that a woman can experience (59). Older women often are faced with the death of an adult child because of sickness or violent death. Often, adult children with a terminal illness will return home to be cared for by their mothers. Thus, the woman's grief will involve not only the loss of the child but the need to deal with the prolonged process of dying associated with the condition.

The loss of a spouse through death or divorce usually will cause psychologic distress (60). Any emotional problems that a woman previously demonstrated may increase in response to a loss (61). Thus, if she is an anxious individual or tends to be depressed, these symptoms usually will become more severe during the grieving process.

A number of situations and grief reactions have been labeled morbid grief because the reaction was abnormal and could, in many cases, have other serious consequences (59). The first morbid grief reaction is a delay in reaction, which usually is seen when the patient is in a life-threatening situation and is unable to grieve appropriately for the loss of a loved one. For example, a husband and a wife are in a car accident in which the husband dies and the wife is seriously injured. This situation may result in the delay of the grief reaction in the wife until she has recovered adequately from her physical injuries. Thus, the full-blown grief reaction may not occur until several months after the accident and may appear inappropriate when it does.

Another morbid grief reaction is the distorted grief reaction. This is frequently seen in an adult daughter who has lost her mother with whom she was very close. She may not show evidence of grief but may take on the mannerisms of the deceased. She may style her hair, dress, and even walk like her deceased mother. If her mother died of an illness, the daughter may even take on the symptoms of the illness that her mother demonstrated. This type of reaction may be prolonged but generally will subside as the individual grieves more normally and returns to her usual behavior pattern. As life expectancy increases, this reaction may be seen more often in older women with aging parents.

Pathologic alterations in relationships frequently are seen in bereaved individuals, leading to altered relationships with friends and relatives. This may occur because the bereaved individual blames friends or relatives, in part, for the death of a loved one or because of guilt.

Inappropriate behavior patterns often are seen in individuals experiencing abnormal grief reactions. These may include inappropriate fears, such as a fear of leaving home, a belief that others are trying to harm them, or a fear of engaging in normal activities, such as driving a car. The bereaved may develop compulsions that require them to act out certain behavior patterns, and they may have difficulty sleeping and may walk the streets at night without any obvious purpose.

An extreme example of morbid grief is the development of psychotic behavior patterns. In this situation, a woman may hear voices instructing her to perform certain commands or she may sit for long periods staring blankly at a wall. This is more common in individuals who have had previous psychotic behavior experiences, but it has been reported in otherwise normal-appearing individuals.

Bereaved individuals may develop an inability to make decisions or take initiative, and this may last 1–2 years after the loss of a loved one. It may be particularly difficult for older individuals and may last longer. In this situation, they may become susceptible to predators who may include individuals who have been close to them. Likewise, another form of abnormal grief is a more active destructiveness. In this case, the grieving individual may carry out actions that may injure her financially, such as signing over her property to children or other family members, and possibly even running away. Although this type of reaction often is seen after a divorce, it also may occur after the death of a spouse.

An additional morbid grief reaction is agitated depression. This is probably the most dangerous of the morbid grief reactions and, although it often is seen in women mourning the loss of a child, it may occur with other losses as well. In this situation, the bereaved individual becomes despondent and agitated. She cannot sleep. Guilt and anger become mixed in her thought process. She may be so depressed that she contemplates suicide.

The grief reaction often is seen with the loss of an organ or body part, particularly one that relates to the self-image of the individual. Depression frequently is a strong component of this reaction. Some investigators have defined four stages of incorporation that a patient must experience before accepting the loss of an important body part: 1) impact, 2) retreat, 3) acknowledgment, and 4) reconstruction. During the impact period, the woman may not even hear that the organ will be removed. She may actually deny that such information was given to her. However, during the retreat aspect, the individual usually tries to find an alternative to the recommendation that has been made to her. Thus, if a hysterectomy is recommended, she may seek a second opinion to find an alternative therapy. This is probably a healthy reaction and should be encouraged. Acknowledgment occurs when the individual accepts the fact that the organ will be removed and then asks many questions about how the procedure will be performed, the type of anesthetic that will be used, and the length of hospital stay. She also may wish to know how she will feel after the operation and the amount of time that she may miss from work and other activities. During the final or reconstruction phase, she will question what she will be like after the procedure and how others will respond to her. In the case of a woman undergoing a hysterectomy, she may wish to know the impact of the procedure on her sexuality and any changes she may expect in how her husband relates to her. It is important to involve both members of the couple in these discussions so that each will know what to expect after the procedure. If a woman goes through the stages appropriately before the procedure is performed, she is less likely to experience depression and grief than if she is rushed into the procedure (62).

For many women, the loss of a job or the inability to perform a physical activity that they have enjoyed also may bring on some form of grief reaction. Encouraging bereaved patients to reach out to others and to develop new activities is an important direction to follow (43). Kindness and support from friends, family, and the medical profession usually is all that is necessary to help a woman through a period of bereavement or loss.

Impending Death

It is particularly important for physicians caring for older women to understand their patients' reactions to impending death. In 1969, an observation was made that death has always been distasteful to individuals and was never considered a possible outcome for their lives (63). It was found that individuals viewed death as a bad event, a frightening happening, and sometimes that death, in itself, called for retribution and punishment.

Five stages through which an individual progresses in the acceptance of the inevitability of death were described: 1) denial, 2) anger, 3) bargaining, 4) depression, and 5) acceptance. The denial stage usually is temporary and is brought about by the shock of learning that one is facing a condition from which she cannot recover. She may not remember that she has been told this, and it may be necessary to repeat the information to her on several occasions. Transition to acceptance may depend on the nature of her illness and the amount of time that she has left before death is expected to occur. It also may depend on the way in which she had prepared herself during her life to cope with a serious illness. As with the loss of an organ, she often will seek second opinions when given such information. This is healthy and should be encouraged.

The next stage is reached when the patient accepts the fact that death will occur in the foreseeable future and usually is represented by anger. She may be difficult to deal with during this period because she may take her anger out on health care workers and family. This behavior may make these individuals less likely to want to deal with her, and this, of course, is the opposite of what she wants. It is best to approach a patient in this stage with understanding and patience.

The next stage is bargaining, when the patient essentially tries to put her life in order. She may rediscover her religious roots and make peace with family members and friends with whom she has quarrelled. She often will put her financial affairs in order and update her will. The bargaining aspect is probably carried out in the hopes of a reprieve. However, she generally will derive mental satisfaction from this stage.

The final stage is acceptance. If the patient lives long enough, she will get to this stage. It has been speculated that the acceptance stage may be simply the wearing down of an individual by the symptoms of a disease and that death may actually be a relief. However, it has been found that many individuals who did not experience severe symptoms achieved acceptance.

Depression may occur at any time, and it may be severe enough to require treatment. This often is related to the woman's personality type and the way she copes with problems.

Everyone will die sooner or later, and physicians need to understand what dying patients are experiencing so that they may be able to treat these individuals with patience and kindness, and, where possible, make the final transition as reasonable as possible. During this process, it is appropriate for the physician to discuss such matters as the need for estate planning, the designation of an executor or an individual with power of attorney, and directions regarding living wills and directives. When necessary, community services, including hospice care, can be considered. At the end of life, palliative care and pain relief should become the physician's primary responsibility to the patient.

 ## Counseling: Establishing a Dialogue

Generally, older individuals have developed excellent social skills that can camouflage their true mental, physical, and emotional well-being. Therefore, physicians can address their well-being by establishing a dialogue through open-ended questions:

- Are there things that you used to do that you no longer feel capable of doing?

- How would you rate your stamina and strength today compared with your strength 1 year or 5 years ago?

- How is your memory?

- Do you find familiar items, such as names and places, difficult to remember?
- Do you make plans for the future?
- Do you enjoy your grandchildren?
- Are you active with social activities, such as church and clubs?
- Do you have a positive outlook on life?

It is important for physicians to be aware of their patients' abilities to care for themselves and their current living conditions. With this information, physicians can counsel their patients, when necessary, about adjustments that can improve the quality of their lives and their environments. It is important for physicians to know the answers to the following questions about their patients:

- Who are her support persons?
- Is she able to live alone, does she require someone living with her, or should she live in an assisted-living facility or a nursing home?
- Is she able to understand the medications that she takes, read the labels and interpret the instructions, and remove the lid from the container?
- Does she use a weekly pill dispenser for her medications to ensure that she takes them and, if she is visually impaired, does she take the correct pills?
- Is she vulnerable to intimidation or abuse?
- Has she experienced a loss or is she experiencing a grief reaction that may be interfering with her daily activities?

In patients with clear disabilities in any of these areas, discussing limitations with a family member or other caregiver may be useful.

Prevention

After evaluating the patient and developing an impression of her abilities and limitations, the physician is able to offer preventive strategies and develop interventions to improve her quality of life, prevent or delay disease states, and perhaps increase her longevity.

In many cases, it may be necessary to promote consultation with other members of the health care team, such as geriatricians, ophthalmologists, dentists, psychologists, psychiatrists, dietitians, exercise therapists, physiotherapists, occupational therapists, nurses, and social workers. However, obstetrician–gynecologists are still in a position to undertake many essential health care needs of older women, and they should encourage preventive and health maintenance practices (Box 5).

Box 5. Preventive and Health Maintenance Practices

Screening and immunization

- Appropriate periodic preventive health processes (eg, mammography, colonoscopy, bone density assessment, hypertension screening, lipid assessment, and screening for diabetes mellitus)
- Appropriate immunizations

Lifestyle modification

- Good dietary habits and nutrition
- Adequate sleep (7–8 hours per night)
- Reasonable exercise
- Smoking cessation
- Decreased alcohol intake

Safety isues

- Seatbelt use
- Use of protective gear during recreational activities
- Use of safe footwear
- Prevention of falls
- Avoidance of inappropriate strenuous tasks and activities

Future planning

- Creation of advance directives
- Designation of health care proxy

Nutrition

A woman's metabolic needs tend to change after menopause, with the cessation of ovarian function. A woman's nutritional needs also may be affected by illness or disease states that can develop as she ages. Appetite may be affected by age-related changes in the senses of taste and smell. Medications also may alter her nutritional state by affecting appetite, metabolism, and absorption or by interfering with the nutrients within her body. In addition, social factors may be in play. If the patient is disabled, she may not be able to get to the store to obtain fresh nutritious ingredients and, therefore, may subsist on a diet of foods that can be stored in bulk. Finally, if the patient has depression or dementia, she may not have the interest or ability to prepare nutritional meals.

Depending on current weight and health status, caloric intake usually should be approximately 1,900 calories per day, or approximately 25 calories/kg, in women older than 50 years. The recommended dietary allowances also decrease in older women (Table 4). Approximately 30% of the recommended caloric intake may be fats, and cholesterol should not exceed 300 mg per day. It also is recommended that the diets of older individuals should consist of 45–50% carbohydrates; 55–60% should be complex carbohydrates. Most foods containing complex carbohydrates also contain vitamins and minerals making them particularly attractive for older women. There is some disagreement about limiting protein in the diets of older women because the studies in nitrogen balance in older individuals have been difficult to reproduce. However, protein stores diminish with age because of a reduction in lean body mass, and there is some disagreement about whether body protein synthesis also is decreased (64). Serum albumen levels decrease with age, and protein metabolism is dependent on kidney function that also may decrease with age. Although these are uncertainties, it has been recommended that older individuals consume 12–14% of their calories as protein, but larger amounts may be needed in those who are undernourished or who may have an illness relating to nitrogen loss (64).

Vitamin deficiencies commonly occur in older individuals for a variety of reasons, which vary from low intake to an increased incidence of atrophic gastritis, pernicious anemia, excessive alcohol

Table 4. Recommended Daily Dietary Allowances for Older Women

Nutrient	Recommended Daily Dietary Allowance
Protein	50 g
Vitamins	
A	700 mg
D	800 international units
E	15 mg
K	90 mg*
C	75 mg
Thiamin	1.1 mg
Riboflavin	1.1 mg
Niacin	14 mg
B_6	1.5 mg
Folate	400 mg
B_{12}	2.4 mg
Pantothenic acid	5 mg
Biotin	30 micrograms
Choline	425 mg
Minerals	
Calcium	1,200 mg*
Phosphorus	700 mg
Magnesium	320 mg
Zinc	8 mg
Iron	8 mg
Iodine	150 mg
Selenium	55 mg

*Recommendation is measured as adequate intake. An adequate intake is set instead of a recommended daily dietary allowance if insufficient evidence is available to determine a recommended daily dietary allowance. The adequate intake is based on observed or experimentally determined estimates of average nutrient intake by a group of healthy individuals.

Data from Institute of Medicine (US). Dietary reference intakes for calcium, phosphorus, magnesium, vitamin D, and fluoride. Washington, DC: National Academy Press; 1997; Institute of Medicine (US). Dietary reference intakes for thiamin, riboflavin, niacin, vitamin B_6, folate, vitamin B_{12}, pantothenic acid, biotin, and choline. Washington, DC: National Academy Press; 1998; Institute of Medicine (US). Dietary reference intakes for vitamin C, vitamin E, selenium, and carotenoids. Washington, DC: National Academy Press; 2000; Institute of Medicine (US). Dietary reference intakes for vitamin A, vitamin K, arsenic, boron, chromium, copper, iodine, iron, manganese, molybdenum, nickel, silicon, vanadium, and zinc. Washington, DC: National Academy Press; 2002.

intake, and interference with absorption or metabolism because of the action of medications. Common deficiencies are in vitamin B_{12}, folic acid, and, most importantly, vitamin D (65). Deficiencies of fat-soluble vitamins usually are less frequent. It is now recognized that vitamin D deficiency is very common in older women, especially those residing in long-term care facilities, and is caused by a combination of decreased dietary intake and decreased sunlight exposure with resultant reduction in synthesis of endogenous vitamin D by the skin. The consequences include increased risk of fractures, muscle weakness, and increased risk of falls. Vitamin D and calcium supplementation are important for older women to help prevent osteoporosis. Women should consume 800 international units per day of vitamin D, and women aged 51 years and older should consume 1,200–1,500 mg per day of calcium (66).

In most older individuals, zinc intake does not meet the recommended daily dietary allowance of 8 mg. Individuals with diabetes mellitus, those who abuse alcohol, and those who take diuretics are at particular risk for zinc deficiency. Zinc deficiency has been associated with anorexia nervosa, taste abnormalities, macular degeneration, T-cell dysfunction, and poor wound healing. Based on animal studies, chromium may play a role in preventing hyperglycemia, hypercholesteremia, and opacities of the cornea, but this information has not been proved in humans.

In older individuals, selenium deficiency has been indirectly associated with cancer, coronary artery disease, and immune system dysfunction. A high prevalence of cancer has been noted in areas where crops are low in selenium, and animal studies have tended to support this finding. In one study, increased serum levels up to 130 ng/mL were associated with a decreased risk of cancer, but results indicated that levels above this concentration may be associated with an increased risk of mortality (67). The recommended daily dietary allowance is 55 mg, and higher doses may lead to toxicity, symptoms of which include a garlic odor on the breath, fingernail changes, and peripheral neuropathy (65).

Iron deficiency is common in older individuals for a number of reasons, including poor absorption. Iron deficiency may lead to anemia, but older individuals also are at risk for bleeding from neoplasia, particularly of the gastrointestinal tract, and this should be considered when an older woman is found to be anemic.

There is some evidence that supplementation of certain vitamins and minerals may have health benefits in older women. Consumption of supplemental amounts of vitamin C, vitamin E, and beta carotene have been reported to be associated with lower rates of coronary artery disease, possibly because of their antioxidant properties, but the results of some studies have been contradictory and failed to report beneficial effects. Vitamin E may have a positive effect on the immune system. Niacin may help reduce serum cholesterol levels.

Exercise

Women of all ages should be encouraged to exercise. Even if they have a chronic illness, exercise may improve symptoms or even arrest the condition. There are three types of exercise in which women should be encouraged to participate: 1) endurance, 2) resistance, and 3) balance training. Endurance training improves the cardiovascular status. This status depends on cardiac output (heart rate × stroke volume) and the ability of the muscle to extract oxygen. Cardiovascular endurance decreases with age at a rate of approximately 1 mm^3 of oxygen per kilogram of body weight per year. Maximum heart rate decreases with age at the rate of approximately 1 heartbeat per year. Whereas physical conditioning usually does not change the decrease in heart rate, it does change cardiovascular endurance. Muscle mass also decreases with age, even in very active individuals, but this decrease is more marked in sedentary individuals (68).

Endurance training is defined as the rhythmic contraction of large muscle groups at a specified heart rate for a specific period. It may be weight-bearing training or non–weight-bearing training. Weight-bearing training has a beneficial effect on bone mass but may have a negative effect on hip, knee, or ankle joints. Thus, the type of endurance exercise should depend on the patient's general health and condition and what she is capable of doing physically. It has been shown that endurance training can improve cardiovascular conditioning by as much as 10–30% depending on how hard the individual exercises and the number of muscle groups involved in the exercise (69).

The American College of Sports Medicine and the American Heart Association recommend that women older than 65 years engage in moderately intense aerobic exercise 30 minutes daily, 5 days per week or vigorously intense aerobic exercise 20 minutes daily, 3 days per week and do 8–10 strength-training exercises, 10–15 repetitions of each exercise, 2–3 times per week (70). Women at risk of falling should perform balance exercises and have a physical activity plan. Both aerobic and muscle-strengthening activities are critical for healthy aging. Moderate-intensity aerobic exercise means working hard at about level-6 intensity on a scale of 1–10, a level that allows an individual to carry on a conversation while exercising. Older women with chronic conditions should develop an activity plan with their physician to manage risks and take therapeutic needs into account. Weight-bearing exercises include walking, jogging, stair climbing, cross-country skiing, and aerobic dance. Non–weight-bearing exercises include swimming, rowing, and upper-body exercises.

Endurance training improves cardiovascular conditioning and generally gives the individual greater energy. Before an older woman embarks on an endurance exercise program, her cardiovascular status should be evaluated so that specific guidelines can be suggested.

The objective of resistance training is to improve muscle mass. Muscles are composed of two types of muscle fibers: 1) slow twitch and 2) fast twitch. The fast-twitch fibers account for rapid and powerful movements, and these tend to decrease in number with age, whereas the slow-twitch fibers remain more stable (68). Weight-lifting exercises help increase the number of fast-twitch fibers and the size of the muscle, thereby increasing muscle strength. Individuals of all ages and condition can perform exercises using weights. They should be performed, at least at the start, under the direction of an exercise expert, such as a personal trainer. Specific muscle groups can be exercised as determined by the patient's needs, or the exercises may be generalized.

Posture and balance training is important for older women because it may decrease falls (69). It also will improve posture. Posture and balance training integrates the sensory and motor systems and helps the individual react more quickly to changes in her environment. Balance training can be broken down into static and dynamic components. Static exercises include balancing the center of gravity or standing in the same spot. The exercises may begin on a wide base but then are performed on progressively narrower bases, going gradually from a double-legged support to a semitandem, to a tandem, to a single-leg support, and to static support on toes. Exercises may be sit-to-stand or cervical spine rotation or twist, side bending, and scapular retraction and elevation. *Dynamic balance* is maintaining the balance during movements. It can be made progressively more difficult by narrowing the base of support and using side steps, crossover steps, forward or backward steps, high steps, heel-to-toe walking, and toe tapping. Aerobic dance and yoga can be useful in carrying out such exercises.

A well-rounded exercise program includes attention to endurance, resistance training, and balance. Aside from the obvious benefits of improving endurance, muscle mass, strength, and balance, many individuals with chronic illness experience an improvement in their symptoms. Pain relief in patients with arthritis has been noted, and patients with high blood pressure, chronic obstructive pulmonary disease, congestive heart failure, pulmonary hypertension, left ventricular dysfunction, angina, and cardiac arrhythmias often experience symptomatic relief.

Immunization

In the United States, immunization recommendations are reviewed regularly and updated by the Advisory Committee on Immunization Practices of the Centers for Disease Control and Prevention (71).

Women aged 50 years and older should be encouraged to obtain an influenza vaccination annually. Vaccination is particularly important for those who are residents in chronic care facilities. It is estimated that approximately 20,000 deaths are caused by influenza in older adults annually in the United States. Because the influenza vaccine has an estimated efficacy of 70% and only 30% of at-risk individuals receive the vaccine, a greater use of the vaccine in older individuals could prevent 9,800 deaths annually (72).

Women aged 65 years and older should be offered pneumococcal vaccination with booster immunization every 5 years after initial immunization in those with risk factors of poor pulmonary function or other chronic illnesses. It is estimated that 40,000 deaths occur annually among older individuals because of pneu-mococcal infection (10). The pneumococcus vaccine has an esti-mated vaccine efficacy of 60%, but only 14% of exposed individuals have been vaccinated. Therefore, it is estimated that 20,640 deaths could be prevented annually if the vaccine was used more widely (72).

All women should receive a tetanus–diphtheria booster. This booster should be given every 10 years.

Hepatitis B virus vaccination should be offered to high-risk older individuals, especially those who are recipients of blood products, live in households with intravenous drug users, or have sexual contact with hepatitis B virus carriers. Dialysis recipients also should be immunized (71). Hepatitis A virus vaccination also is recommended for high-risk older adults, especially those who travel outside the United States.

Inactivated polio vaccination should be offered to older indi-viduals who have never been vaccinated or whose vaccination was received many years ago and who require a booster shot. This immunization is important for those who interact with young children who may have been given the oral polio vaccine (live vaccine) recently or for those who travel to countries where polio is still a problem.

The newly developed shingles vaccine is now recommended for individuals older than 60 years who have had chicken pox. This vaccine has been shown to reduce the risk of shingles in older individuals by approximately 50%.

Older individuals who travel outside the United States should be adequately immunized for diseases that may be prevalent in the areas to which they are traveling. In such situations, it is best to consult the Centers for Disease Control and Prevention or a travel clinic to determine which immunizations are recommended. Such individuals should be offered malaria prophylaxis if they are planning trips to areas where malaria is prevalent (71).

Safety Precautions

Most safety issues are common sense, but they often are not con-sidered as carefully as they should be. The annual health mainte-nance visit is a good time to remind older patients of safety issues regarding the use of safety belts while traveling in vehicles, the use of protective gear for recreational activities, avoidance of strenuous exercise, and storage of firearms in the home.

The national media and most state laws have emphasized the need for using safety belts while traveling in vehicles, yet older individuals often do not use safety belts because many were raised at a time when safety belts were not present in vehicles. It is important to stress the need for safety belt use, especially because most states now have penalties for not wearing safety belts.

Many active older individuals ride bicycles, horses, and motorcycles, and some roller skate or ice skate. Use of protective gear, including helmets, knee pads, and elbow pads, to prevent head and limb injuries during these activities should be emphasized.

It is important to stress that inappropriate and strenuous exercises should be avoided. Although exercise is excellent for older individuals, pushing the body to extreme fatigue may challenge a compromised cardiovascular system. It also may cause bone and joint pain and injury. Generally, safe tasks and activities should be encouraged. Activities that may pose possible risk should be avoided.

Determining the presence of firearms in the household is important. It has been estimated that there are firearms in 70% of American households. If firearms are present in the household, the individuals with access to them should be aware of safety precautions. Firearms should be stored unloaded, and they should be kept locked up. As with many other issues, asking patients about firearms may yield information about the patients' living conditions of which the physician is unaware.

Considerations for Medical Management

There are unique considerations in the medical management of older patients. It is important for obstetrician–gynecologists to be aware of the interaction of different medications and the risks and benefits of the use of hormone therapy when treating these patients.

Drug Interactions

Many older patients take multiple drugs on a daily basis. Multiple drug therapy creates an opportunity for drug interactions. Also, older individuals may have an increased vulnerability to drugs because they metabolize or excrete drugs differently than younger individuals and because physiologic changes in older individuals may lead to poor or accelerated absorption of some drugs (73). Drug interactions often occur in older individuals and may lead to hospitalization for drug toxicity. Researchers reported a sixfold increase in admissions for hypoglycemia in older patients taking glyburide who were subsequently treated with cotrimoxazole in the previous week (74). They also noted a 12-fold increase in admissions from digoxin toxicity if the patient had been subsequently treated with clarithromycin. Patients taking angiotensin-converting enzyme inhibitors had a 20-fold increase in admission for hyperkalemia if they were treated with a potassium-sparing diuretic. Approximately 12% of women older than 65 years who begin taking selective serotonin reuptake inhibitors will develop hyponatremia, which may be considerably symptomatic, within the first 2 weeks of treatment.

Older individuals may use drugs improperly because of hearing loss, which makes it difficult for them to understand instructions; visual impairments, which make it difficult for them to read instructions or drug labels correctly; or memory loss, which makes it difficult for them to remember how or when to take their medication or whether they have taken it. For all of these reasons, physicians may have a more difficult time obtaining compliance and appropriate drug response in older patients.

Problems with drug absorption occur for a number of reasons, including loss of acidic gastric fluid pH; slower gastric emptying time; decreased intestinal mobility; decreased gastrointestinal fluid secretion, including volume and composition; decreased or compromised gastrointestinal blood flow; gastrointestinal disease; and general health problems. Drug distribution in the body also is an important issue. Total body water and blood volume and lean body mass (ie, muscle tissue) tend to decrease with age. There is a relative increase in body fat, from 18% to 36% of total body weight in men and from 33% to 45% of total body weight in women. Thus, drugs that are readily soluble in fat are more readily stored in older patients, and to a greater extent in women than in men. A drug that is stored in fat would have a greater volume of distribution and, when a single dose is administered, it would have a lower plasma volume compared with drugs that are not readily stored in fat (75).

Another important feature is drug metabolism. Liver size and blood flow decrease with age. Thus, drugs that are metabolized in the liver are cleared more slowly and have a longer plasma half-life. For some drugs, the plasma half-life is increased as much as 75% in older women (73).

The use of drugs that are excreted by the kidney may be an additional concern for older women. Beginning in the fourth decade of life, changes in renal blood flow, glomerular filtration rate, and active tubular secretion and absorption begin to occur. Kidney function decreases with age, and drugs that are eliminated by the kidney show an increased plasma half-life and a decreased clearance rate (76).

Because of all of these previously mentioned factors, older individuals generally are sensitive or more responsive to drugs than younger adults. In some situations, however, older individuals are less responsive to certain drugs. For example, higher doses of the β-adrenergic blocker, propanolol, are required to obtain the desired physiologic effect in older individuals. This may occur because cardiac β-receptors are less sensitive in older individuals (77).

Some commonly used medications show increased sensitivity in older individuals. Some drugs, such as the benzodiazepines, can cause depression at lower dosage levels in older individuals. In these cases, the drug plasma levels at which depression occurs are inversely related to age. Researchers studied individuals being prepared for dental or endoscopic procedures (78). They found that patients aged 80 years or older required an average dose of 10 mg of diazepam compared with 30 mg for patients aged 20 years and that plasma levels required for sedation in individuals older than 80 years were one third to one half the amount required for younger individuals. Similarly, older patients are more sensitive to warfarin (79). Because patients in this age group often require anticoagulation, this sensitivity must be taken into consideration.

Although not life-threatening, many drugs, such as antihypertensive drugs, may have adverse effects on sexual performance and urinary and bowel function. Central sympatholytics, β-adrenergic blockers, α-adrenergic blockers, and thiazide diuretics frequently impair sexual performance. Many of the psychotropic drugs and other frequently used drugs, such as cimetidine and metoclopramide, can cause sexual dysfunction. Anticholinergic drugs may be associated with decreased libido and even impotence in men.

Some older individuals are more susceptible to parkinsonian-like symptoms induced by neuroleptics, antiemetics, methyldopa, reserpine, and diazepam (80). Because drug interactions may occur, physicians must carefully choose the medications that they prescribe for older patients, keeping in mind that one drug may change the rate of absorption and enhance the bioavailability of another drug. A drug may increase or decrease the rate of metabolism. A drug also may decrease the rate of excretion of another drug, or a drug may influence the protein binding of another drug. In addition, drug absorption may be affected by binding within the gastrointestinal tract, changes in the stomach pH, a decrease in gastrointestinal mobility, changes in intestinal flora, and alteration of drug metabolism within the wall of the intestine.

It is suggested that physicians caring for older individuals obtain detailed drug histories of their older patients, including all medications currently taken (prescription, nonprescription, and alternative therapy). It is best to have the patient bring all medications to her annual health visit. Physicians should prescribe only drugs for which there is a clear need and where the chance of benefit clearly outweighs the risk of adverse effects. The patient should be aware of the goals of therapy and the need for medication and should clearly understand how the medication is to be administered. The patient should be asked for feedback on her response to the drug with emphasis on adverse effects. Whenever possible, a family member should be included so that the instructions are clearly understood and the need for feedback is met. Patients should be evaluated frequently and carefully to ensure that the desired effect of the drug is being realized and that adverse effects are not present. If the patient experiences adverse effects, the value of continuing the drug must be considered. For older patients, lower doses should always be prescribed first and given in small increments at longer intervals than would be prescribed for younger patients. If the patient has difficulty swallowing tablets, liquid preparations may be substituted.

The patient should be given written instructions for using the medication, and the physician should verify that she can read and understand the instructions. The physician also should make sure that the patient can open the drug container and read the label. The patient should know the reason for the use of each drug. Whenever possible, the physician should use a once-per-day dosage schedule and help the patient establish a daily schedule so that she will know if she has taken the drug. The use of weekly pill containers may be helpful. If necessary, plasma drug levels can be used to determine the appropriate drug dosage and the interval between dosages. An experienced pharmacist may be helpful in many of these situations.

Hormone Therapy

Epidemiologic data have suggested a possible increase in the risk of breast cancer in women using hormone therapy with progestins. Hormone therapy also is associated with an increased risk of thromboembolism and stroke and a possible increase in the risk of coronary artery disease in certain women (81). However, frail women with osteopenia or osteoporosis may benefit greatly from hormone therapy, whereas obese, robust women may not. The care of each patient must be individualized and her risks and benefits estimated. The use of hormone therapy should be based on the physician's estimate of the benefits that the patient would derive and the patient's level of comfort with the possible risks. In this way, each patient is treated as an individual, her needs and risks are properly assessed, and she is able to make a well-informed decision about the use of hormone therapy.

 Complementary and Alternative Medicine

Increasingly, patients are seeking therapies with complementary and alternative medicine. Several of these therapies may be helpful to older women for a variety of conditions.

Older individuals experience many aches and pains that may not have serious pathologic causes but that may be relieved or improved by massage therapy and acupuncture. Referral to practitioners in these areas for these purposes is reasonable.

The use of ginkgo biloba as treatment for memory loss is a popular alternative therapy. However, a recent double-masked study demonstrated no value of the use of this herb in improving cognition in otherwise healthy older adults (82). Most herbal remedies marketed today have not been tested in this fashion.

The use of dehydroepiandrosterone sulfate was studied for 2 years in 57 elderly women with low serum dehydroepiandrosterone sulfate concentrations in a double-blind, placebo-controlled trial. No significant effect was noted on body composition measurements, peak volume of oxygen consumption per minute, muscle strength, or insulin insensitivity (83). In another study, therapy with the use of dehydroepiandrosterone sulfate for 6 months significantly reduced visceral and subcutaneous fat in 28 elderly women as noted on magnetic resonance imaging (84). This finding suggests that therapy with this agent might have a positive effect in preventing atherosclerosis. Clearly, further study is indicated.

Physicians should caution patients about using agents in which efficacy is untested. In addition, many complementary and alternative therapies use agents that have relatively strong physiologic activity and may interact with other medications the patient may be taking. Thus, when patients decide to use alternative medical preparations, they should be advised of the potential for interaction with current prescribed medications.

Summary

The obstetrician–gynecologist is well suited to continue caring for women during the later period of their lives. Care should consist of a holistic approach to the woman and should address her physical, emotional, and psychosocial needs. An awareness of conditions that are more common in older women and knowledge of current screening recommendations are important tools obstetrician–gynecologists can use to help older patients prevent disease, prolong their lives, and improve their quality of life.

Resources

American College of Obstetricians and Gynecologists

Resource Kit

Domestic Elder Abuse: Practical Tools for Providers
of Women's Health Care (AA400)

Patient Education Materials

A Healthy Lifestyle for Women Ages 65 and Older (AB019)

Reducing Your Risk of Cancer (AP007)

Pelvic Support Problems (AP012)

Pain During Intercourse (AP020)

The Menopause Years (AP047)

Osteoporosis (AP048)

Hormone Therapy (AP066)

Mammography (AP076)

Urinary Incontinence (AP081)

Immunizations for Adolescents and Adults (AP117)

Keeping Your Heart Healthy (AP122)

Managing High Blood Pressure (AP123)

Bowel Control Problems (AP139)

Herbal Products for Menopause (AP158)

Menopausal Bleeding (AP 162)

Surgery for Urinary Incontinence (AP166)

American College of Obstetricians and Gynecologists' WebTreats

Aging
www.acog.org/departments/dept._notice.cfm?recno =
20&bulletin = 4534

Menopause
www.acog.org/departments/dept._notice.cfm?recno =
20&bulletin = 2548

Agencies and Organizations

American Geriatrics Society
The Empire State Building
350 Fifth Avenue, Suite 801
New York, NY 10118
Tel: (212) 308-1414
Fax: (212) 832-8646
E-mail: info@americangeriatrics.org
Web: www.americangeriatrics.org

(continued)

Resources *(continued)*

Agencies and Organizations *(continued)*

American Psychological Association
750 First Street NE
Washington, DC 20002-4242
Tel: (800) 374-2721
    (202) 336-5500
Web: www.apa.org

National Institute on Aging
Building 31, Room 5C27
31 Center Drive, MSC 2292
Bethesda, MD 20892
Tel: (800) 222-2225
    (301) 496-1752
Fax: (301) 496-1072
E-mail: niainfo@mail.nih.gov
Web: www.nia.nih.gov
       www.nia.nih.gov/HealthInformation/Publications/falls.htm
       (Age Page: Fractures and Falls)

📖 Test Your Clinical Skills

Complete the answer sheet at the back of this book and return it to ACOG to receive Continuing Medical Education credits. The answers appear on page 63.

Directions: Select the one best answer or completion.

1. Drug therapy should be started in a postmenopausal woman with coronary artery disease when LDL cholesterol first exceeds
   A. 100 mg/dL
   B. 130 mg/dL
   C. 160 mg/dL
   D. 190 mg/dL

2. How often should women older than 35 years be screened for hypothyroidism?
   A. Annually
   B. Every 3 years
   C. Every 5 years
   D. Every 10 years

3. Which of the following actions is precipitated through the neurotransmitter acetylcholine?
   A. Contraction of lower urethra
   B. Contraction of lower bladder neck
   C. Relaxation of upper bladder
   D. Relaxation of upper urethra

4. Interest in which of the following sexual activities has been reported to increase among older individuals?
   A. Masturbation level in women
   B. Masturbation level in men
   C. Interest in mutual masturbation
   D. Interest in intercourse

5. Older individuals who take diuretics are at increased risk of deficiency of
   A. vitamin D
   B. folic acid
   C. selenium
   D. zinc

6. The amount of moderately intense exercise recommended by the American College of Sports Medicine is
   A. 30 minutes, 7 days per week
   B. 30 minutes, 5 days per week
   C. 30 minutes, 3 days per week
   D. 60 minutes, 3 days per week

7. An example of non–weight-bearing exercise is
   A. walking
   B. stair climbing
   C. dancing
   D. rowing

8. Which of the following vaccines is only recommended for older individuals at high risk?
   A. Influenza
   B. Pneumococcal
   C. Hepatitis B
   D. Tetanus

9. Older individuals have decreased sensitivity to which of the following drugs?
   A. Diazepam
   B. Propanolol
   C. Warfarin
   D. Benzodiazepines

10. Three months after the death of her mother, a 62-year-old woman begins exclusively wearing her mother's dresses. This is an example of which type of morbid grief reaction?
    A. Delayed
    B. Distorted
    C. Compulsive
    D. Psychotic

11. When a patient who has been reluctant to agree to a needed hysterectomy asks questions about how her sexual function will change, she is probably in which stage of incorporation?
    A. Impact
    B. Retreat
    C. Acknowledgment
    D. Reconstruction

12. A 48-year-old woman has been told by a surgeon and an oncologist that she has terminal breast cancer. She wants another opinion. This behavior is most often seen in which of the five stages of the acceptance of the inevitability of death?
    A. Denial
    B. Anger
    C. Bargaining
    D. Acceptance

13. Studies of dehydroepiandrosterone therapy produced which of the following results?
    A. Increased muscle strength
    B. Increased insulin sensitivity
    C. Decreased libido
    D. Decreased subcutaneous fat

References

1. Heron M. Deaths: leading causes for 2004. Natl Vital Stat Rep 2007;56:1–95. (Level III)

2. Martin GM. Segmental and unimodal progeroid syndromes of man. In: Harrison DE, editor. Genetic effects on aging II. Caldwell (NJ): Telford Press; 1990. p. 493–520. (Level III)

3. Harman D. Free radical theory of aging: role of free radicals in the origination and evolution of life, aging, and disease processes. In: Johnson JE, Walford R, Harman D, Miquel J, editors. Free radicals, aging, and degenerative diseases. New York (NY): Allen R. Liss, 1986. p. 3–49. (Level III)

4. Reid TM, Loeb LA. Tandem double CC to TT mutations are produced by reactive oxygen species. Proc Natl Acad Sci U S A 1993;90:3904–7. (Level III)

5. Cerami A, Vlassara H, Brownlee M. Glucose and aging. Sci Am 1987;256: 90–6. (Level III)

6. Martin GM, Sprague CA, Norwood TH, Pendergrass WR, Bornstein P, Hoehn H, et al. Do hyperplastoid cell lines "differentiate themselves to death"? In: Cristofalo VJ, Holeckova E, editors. Cell impairment in aging and development. Advances in Experimental Medicine and Biology; vol. 53. New York (NY): Plenum Press; 1975. p. 67–90. (Level III)

7. Walston J, Hadley EC, Ferrucci L, Guralnik JM, Newman AB, Studenski, et al. Research agenda for frailty in older adults: toward a better understanding of physiology and etiology: summary from the American Geriatrics Society/National Institute on Aging Research Conference on Frailty in Older Adults. J Am Geriatr Soc 2006;54:991–1001. (Level III)

8. Katz S, Ford AB, Moskowitz RW, Jackson BA, Jaffe MW. Studies of illness in the aged. The index of ADL: a standardized measure of biological and psychosocial function. JAMA 1963;185:914–9. (Level III)

9. Lawton MP, Brody EM. Assessment of older people: self-maintaining and instrumental activities of daily living. Gerontologist 1969;9:179–86. (Level III)

10. Primary and preventive care: periodic assessments. ACOG Committee Opinion No. 357. American College of Obstetricians and Gynecologists. Obstet Gynecol 2006:108:1615–22. (Level III)

11. American Academy of Ophthalmology. Comprehensive adult medical eye evaluation. Preferred Practice Pattern. San Francisco (CA): AAO; 2005. (Level III)

12. Executive Summary of The Third Report of The National Cholesterol Education Program (NCEP) Expert Panel on Detection, Evaluation, and Treatment of High Blood Cholesterol in Adults (Adult Treatment Panel III). Expert Panel on Detection, Evaluation, and Treatment of High Blood Cholesterol in Adults. JAMA 2001;285:2486–97. (Level III)

13. Chobanian AV, Bakris GL, Black HR, Cushman WC, Green LA, Izzo JL Jr, et al. The Seventh Report of the Joint National Committee on Prevention,

Detection, Evaluation, and Treatment of High Blood Pressure: the JNC 7 report. National Heart, Lung, and Blood Institute Joint National Committee on Prevention, Detection, Evaluation, and Treatment of High Blood Pressure; National High Blood Pressure Education Program Coordinating Committee [published erratum appears in JAMA 2003;290:197]. JAMA 2003;289: 2560–72. (Level III)

14. Blair SN, Goodyear NN, Gibbons LW, Cooper KH. Physical fitness and incidence of hypertension in healthy normotensive men and women. JAMA 1984;252:487–90. (Level II-3)

15. Prevention of stroke by antihypertensive drug treatment in older persons with isolated systolic hypertension. Final results of the Systolic Hypertension in the Elderly Program (SHEP). SHEP Cooperative Research Group. JAMA 1991;265:3255–64. (Level I)

16. Centers for Disease Prevention and Control. National diabetes fact sheet: general information and national estimates on diabetes in the United States, 2007. Atlanta (GA): CDC; 2008. Available at: www.cdc.gov/diabetes/pubs/pdf/ndfs_2007.pdf. Retrieved February 6, 2009. (Level III)

17. Robuschi G, Safran M, Braverman LE, Gnudi A, Roti E. Hypothyroidism in the elderly. Endocrine Rev 1987;8:142–53. (Level III)

18. Ladenson PW, Singer PA, Ain KB, Bagchi N, Bigos ST, Levy EG, et al. American Thyroid Association guidelines for detection of thyroid dysfunction [published erratum appears in Arch Intern Med 2001;161:284]. Arch Intern Med 2000;160:1573–5. (Level III)

19. Griffin MA, Solomon DH. Hyperthyroidism in the elderly. J Am Geriatr Soc 1986;34:887–92. (Level III)

20. Miller M. Disorders of the thyroid. In: Tallis R, Fillit H, Brocklehurst JC, editors. Brocklehurst's textbook of geriatric medicine and gerontology, 6th ed. London: Churchill Livingstone; 2003. p. 1165–83. (Level III)

21. Seligman PA. Hematologic problems. In: Jahnigen DW, Schrier RW, editors. Geriatric medicine. 2nd ed. Cambridge (MA): Blackwell Science; 1996. p. 781–8. (Level III)

22. Andresen SW. Geriatric oncology. In: Jahnigen DW, Schrier RW, editors. Geriatric medicine. 2nd ed. Cambridge (MA): Blackwell Science; 1996. p. 789–805. (Level III)

23. Riggs BL, Melton LJ, 3rd. Involutional osteoporosis. N Engl J Med 1986;314: 1676–86. (Level III)

24. Osteoporosis. ACOG Practice Bulletin No. 50. American College of Obstetricians and Gynecologists. Obstet Gynecol 2004;103:203–16. (Level III)

25. Beckett WS. Epidemiology and etiology of lung cancer. Clin Chest Med 1993;14:1–15. (Level III)

26. Berman BA, Gritz ER. Women and smoking: current trends and issues for the 1990s. J Subst Abuse 1991;3:221–38. (Level III)

27. Jemal A, Siegel R, Ward E, Hao Y, Xu J, Murray T, et al. Cancer statistics, 2008. CA Cancer J Clin 2008;58:71–96. (Level II-3)

28. Cervical cytology screening. ACOG Practice Bulletin No. 45. American College of Obstetricians and Gynecologists. Obstet Gynecol 2003;102:417–27. (Level III)

29. American Cancer Society. Cancer facts and figures 2008. Atlanta (GA): ACS; 2008. (Level II-3)

30. U.S. Preventive Services Task Force. Screening for cervical cancer. Guide to clinical preventive services. 3rd ed. Rockville (MD): Agency for Healthcare Research and Quality; 2003. p. 277–85. (Level III)

31. Feuer EJ, Wun LM, Boring CC, Flanders WD, Timmel MJ, Tong T. The lifetime risk of developing breast cancer. J Natl Cancer Inst 1993;85:892–7. (Level III)

32. Black JS, Sefcik T, Kapoor W. Health promotion and disease prevention in the elderly. Comparison of house staff and attending physician attitudes and practices. Arch Intern Med 1990;150:389–93. (Level III)

33. Breast cancer screening. ACOG Practice Bulletin No. 42. American College of Obstetricians and Gynecologists. Obstet Gynecol 2003;101:821–31. (Level III)

34. Goff BA, Mandel LS, Drescher CW, Urban N, Gough S, Schurman KM, et al. Development of an ovarian cancer symptom index: possibilities for earlier detection. Cancer 2007;109:221–7. (Level II-2)

35. Winawer SJ, Miller DG, Sherlock P. Risk and screening for colorectal cancer. Adv Intern Med 1984;30:471–96. (Level III)

36. Colonoscopy and colorectal cancer screening and prevention. ACOG Committee Opinion No. 384. American College of Obstetricians and Gynecologists. Obstet Gynecol 2007;110:1199–202. (Level III)

37. Fitzpatrick TB, Sober AJ. Sunlight and skin cancer [editorial]. N Engl J Med 1985;313:818–20. (Level III)

38. American College of Obstetricians and Gynecologists. Intimate partner violence and domestic violence. Special issues in women's health. Washington, DC: ACOG; 2004. p. 169–88. (Level III)

39. Giordano NH, Giordano JA. Elder abuse: a review of the literature. Soc Work 1984;29:232–6. (Level III)

40. Barrett JE, Barrett JA, Oxman TE, Gerber PD. The prevalence of psychiatric disorders in a primary care practice. Arch Gen Psychiatry 1988;45:1100–6. (Level III)

41. Regier DA, Myers JK, Kramer M, Robins LN, Blazer DG, Hough RL, et al. The NIMH Epidemiologic Catchment Area program. Historical context, major objectives, and study population characteristics. Arch Gen Psychiatry 1984; 41:934–41. (Level III)

42. American Psychiatric Association. Diagnostic and statistical manual of mental disorders: DSM-IV-TR. 4th ed., text rev. ed. Washington, DC: APA; 2000. (Level III)

43. Walker EA. Depression, dementia, and delirium. In: Stenchever MA, editor. Health care for the older woman. New York (NY): Chapman & Hall; 1996. p.265–78. (Level III)

44. Hy LX, Keller DM. Prevalence of AD among whites: a summary by levels of severity. Neurology 2000;55:198–204. (Level III)

45. Leslie DL, Marcantonio ER, Zhang Y, Leo-Summers L, Inouye SK. One-year health care costs associated with delirium in the elderly population. Arch Intern Med 2008;168:27–32. (Level III)

46. Centers for Disease Prevention and Control. Falls among older adults: an overview. Atlanta (GA): CDC; 2008. Available at: www.cdc.gov/ncipc/fact sheets/adultfalls.htm. Retrieved February 6, 2009. (Level III)

47. Centers for Disease Prevention and Control. Hip fractures among older adults. Atlanta (GA): CDC; 2008. Available at: www.cdc.gov/ncipc/fact sheets/adulthipfx.htm. Retrieved February 6, 2009. (Level III)

48. Tinetti ME. Clinical practice. Preventing falls in elderly persons. N Engl J Med 2003;348:42–9. (Level III)

49. Gates S, Fisher JD, Cooke MW, Carter YH, Lamb SE. Multifactorial assessment and targeted intervention for preventing falls and injuries among older people in community and emergency care settings: systematic review and meta-analysis. BMJ 2008;336:130–3. (Meta-analysis)

50. Thom D. Variation in estimates of urinary incontinence prevalence in the community: effects of differences in definition, population characteristics, and study type. J Am Geriatr Soc 1998;46:473–80. (Level III)

51. Ouslander JG, Schnelle JF. Incontinence in the nursing home. Ann Intern Med 1995;122:438–49. (Level III)

52. Warshaw GA, Moore JT, Friedman SW, Currie CT, Kennie DC, Kane WJ, et al. Functional disability in the hospitalized elderly. JAMA 1982;248:847–50. (Level III)

53. Brecher EM. Love, sex, and aging: a Consumers Union report. 1st ed. Boston (MA): Little Brown; 1984. (Level III)

54. Cutler WB, Garcia CR, McCoy N. Perimenopausal sexuality. Arch Sex Behav 1987;16:225–34. (Level III)

55. Hawton K, Gath D, Day A. Sexual function in a community sample of middle-aged women with partners: effects of age, marital, socioeconomic, psychiatric, gynecological, and menopausal factors. Arch Sex Behav 1994;23: 375–95. (Level II-3)

56. Masters WH, Johnson VE. Human sexual response. 1st ed. Boston (MA): Little Brown and Company; 1966. (Level III)

57. Heiman JR. Sexuality and aging. In: Stenchever MA, editor. Health care for the older woman. New York (NY): Chapman & Hall; 1996. p. 375–87. (Level III)

58. Quackenbush J. The death of a pet. How it can affect owners. Vet Clin North Am Small Anim Pract 1985;15:395–402. (Level III)

59. Lindemann E. Symptomatology and management of acute grief. Am J Psychiatry 1944;101:141–8. (Level III)

60. Holmes TH, Rahe H. The Social Readjustment Rating Scale. J Psychosom Res 1967;11:213–8. (Level III)

61. Gallagher DE, Breckenridge JN, Thompson LW, Peterson JA. Effects of bereavement on indicators of mental health in elderly widows and widowers. J Gerontol 1983;38:565–71. (Level II-3)

62. Drummond J, Field PA. Emotional and sexual sequelae following hysterectomy. Health Care Women Int 1984;5:261–71. (Level III)

63. Kubler-Ross E. On death and dying. New York (NY): Collier–MacMillan; 1969. (Level III)

64. Fukagawa NK, Young VR. Protein and amino acid metabolism and requirements in older persons. Clin Geriatr Med 1987;3:329–41. (Level III)

65. Morley JE, Mooradian AD, Silver AJ, Heber D, Alfin-Slater RB. Nutrition in the elderly. Ann Intern Med 1988;109:890–904. (Level III)

66. Wicherts IS, van Schoor NM, Boeke AJ, Visser M, Deeg DJ, Smit J, et al. Vitamin D status predicts physical performance and its decline in older persons. J Clin Endocrinol Metab 2007;92:2058–65. (Level II-2)

67. Bleys J, Navas-Acien A, Guallar E. Serum selenium levels and all-cause, cancer, and cardiovascular mortality among U.S. adults. Arch Intern Med 2008;168:404–10. (Level III)

68. Cress ME, Green FA. Exercise and aging: physical fitness. In: Stenchever MA, editor. Health care for the older woman. New York (NY): Chapman and Hall; 1996. p. 69–84. (Level III)

69. Corbin D, Metal-Corbin J. Reach for it! A handbook of health, exercise, and dance activities for older adults. 3rd ed. Peosta (IA): Eddie Bowers Publishing; 1997. (Level III)

70. Nelson ME, Rejeski WJ, Blair SN, Duncan PW, Judge JO, King AC, et al. Physical activity and public health in older adults: recommendation from the American College of Sports Medicine and the American Heart Association. American College of Sports Medicine; American Heart Association. Circulation 2007;116:1094–105. (Level III)

71. Recommended adult immunization schedule: United States, 2009. Advisory Committee on Immunization Practices. Ann Intern Med 2009;150:40–4. (Level III)

72. Gardner P, Schaffner W. Immunization of adults. N Engl J Med 1993;328:1252–8. (Level III)

73. O'Malley K, Crooks J, Duke E, Stevenson IH. Effect of age and sex on human drug metabolism. Br Med J 1971;3:607–9. (Level II-3)

74. Juurlink DN, Mamdani M, Kopp A, Laupacis A, Redelmeier DA. Drug-drug interactions among elderly patients hospitalized for drug toxicity. JAMA 2003;289:1652–8. (Level III)

75. Novak LP. Aging, total body potassium, fat-free mass, and cell mass in males and females between ages 18 and 85 years. J Gerontol 1972;27: 438–43. (Level III)

76. Miller M. Fluid and electrolyte homeostasis in the elderly: physiological changes of ageing and clinical consequences. Baillieres Clin Endocrinol Metab 1997;11:367–87. (Level III)

77. Vestal RE, Wood AJ, Shand DG. Reduced beta-adrenoceptor sensitivity in the elderly. Clin Pharmacol Ther 1979;26:181–6. (Level III)

78. Cook PJ, Flanagan R, James IM. Diazepam tolerance: effect of age, regular sedation, and alcohol. Br Med J (Clin Res Ed) 1984;289:351–3. (Level III)

79. Shepherd AM, Hewick DS, Moreland TA, Stevenson IH. Age as a determinant of sensitivity to warfarin. Br J Clin Pharmacol 1977;4:315–20. (Level III)

80. Wilson JA, MacLennan WJ. Review: drug-induced parkinsonism in elderly patients. Age Aging 1989;18:208–10. (Level III)

81. Rossouw JE, Anderson GL, Prentice RL, LaCroix AZ, Kooperberg C, Stefanick ML, et al. Risks and benefits of estrogen plus progestin in healthy postmenopausal women: principal results from the Women's Health Initiative randomized controlled trial. Writing Group for the Women's Health Initiative Investigators. JAMA 2002;288:321–33. (Level I)

82. Solomon PR, Adams F, Silver A, Zimmer J, DeVeaux R. Gingko for memory enhancement: a randomized controlled trial. JAMA 2002;288:835–40. (Level I)

83. Nair KS, Rizza RA, O'Brien P, Dhatariya K, Short KR, Nehra A, et al. DHEA in elderly women and DHEA and testosterone in elderly men. N Engl J Med 2006;355:1647–59. (Level III)

84. Villareal DT, Holloszy JO. Effect of DHEA on abdominal fat and insulin action in elderly women and men. a randomized controlled trial. JAMA 2004;292: 2243–8. (Level I)

Studies were reviewed and evaluated for quality according to the method outlined by the U.S. Preventive Services Task Force:

I   Evidence obtained from at least one properly designed random-ized controlled trial.

II-1 Evidence obtained from well-designed controlled trials without randomization.

II-2 Evidence obtained from well-designed cohort or case–control analytic studies, preferably from more than one center or research group.

II-3 Evidence obtained from multiple time series with or without the intervention. Dramatic results in uncontrolled experiments also could be regarded as this type of evidence.

III Opinions of respected authorities, based on clinical experience, descriptive studies, or reports of expert committees.

Answers

1. B, 2. C, 3. D, 4. C, 5. D, 6. B, 7. D, 8. C, 9. B, 10. B, 11. D, 12. A, 13. D

Index

Forthcoming Titles

Each monograph in *Clinical Updates in Women's Health Care* is an overview of a topic of importance to obstetrician–gynecologists in practice. Upcoming titles include:

- Migraine and Other Headache Disorders
- Anorectal Disorders

Back issues of published titles are available (for a complete list of titles, visit www.clinicalupdates.org):

- *Eating Disorders* (Volume VII, Number 1, January 2008)
- *Cosmetic Surgery* (Volume VII, Number 2, April 2008)
- *Vision Disorders* (Volume VII, Number 3, July 2008)
- *Lower Urinary Tract Disorders* (Volume VII, Number 4, October 2008)
- *Mood and Anxiety Disorders* (Volume VII, Number 5, November 2008)
- *Polycystic Ovary Syndrome* (Volume VIII, Number 1, January 2009)
- *Vulvar Disorders* (Volume VIII, Number 2, April 2009)
- *Elder Abuse* (Volume VIII, Number 3, July 2009)

You can sign up for a 1-year subscription to *Clinical Updates in Women's Health Care* at the rate of $49 for ACOG members ($95 nonmembers). Individual copies also can be purchased for $20 ($30 nonmembers). You can subscribe by calling (800) 762-2264 or online at sales.acog.org. Online access is available to subscribers at www.clinicalupdates.org.

The Editorial Board welcomes comments and suggestions for topics. Please contact them in care of ACOG Publications (publication@acog.org).

CLINICAL UPDATES
IN WOMEN'S HEALTH CARE

Care of Aging Women
Volume VIII, Number 4, October 2009

Test Your Clinical Skills—and Earn CME Credits

ACCME Accreditation
The American College of Obstetricians and Gynecologists (ACOG) is accredited by the Accreditation Council for Continuing Medical Education (ACCME) to provide continuing medical education for physicians.

AMA PRA Category 1 Credit™ and ACOG Cognate Credit
The American College of Obstetricians and Gynecologists (ACOG) designates this educational activity for a maximum of 5 AMA PRA Category 1 Credit(s)™ or up to a maximum of 5 Category 1 ACOG cognate credit(s). Physicians should only claim credit commensurate with the extent of their participation in the activity.

Actual time spent completing this activity (you may record up to 5 hours):_____.

To obtain credits, complete and return this answer sheet to the address shown below (only original answer sheets will be accepted for credit) or submit your answers online at www.clinicalupdates.org:

1. _____	6. _____	11. _____
2. _____	7. _____	12. _____
3. _____	8. _____	13. _____
4. _____	9. _____	
5. _____	10. _____	

ACOG ID Number __ __ __ __ __ __ __ __ __ __

Name _____

Address _____

City/State/Zip_____

ACOG
Cognate Department
409 12th Street, SW
PO Box 96920
Washington, DC 20090-6920

Reliable Take-Home Information for Your Patients

ACOG Patient Education Pamphlets are designed to complement and supplement the information and advice you provide in the office. After you talk to your older patients, ensure they have accurate information they can refer to and share with their families and friends when they are home.

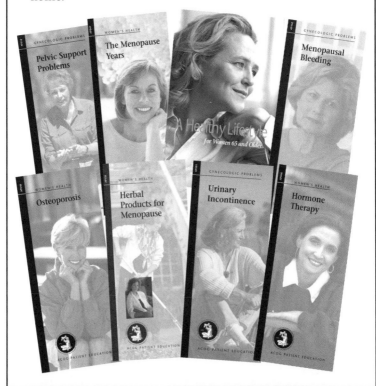